Living in Our
Toxic World

Protect yourself and your family from environmental toxins and reduce your risk of cancer and chronic disease.

Janet L. Black, RN, FNP, MSN, MPH

Peaceful Heart Press

Disclaimer: While the author and publisher have used their best efforts in preparing this book, they make no representations or warranties with respect to the accuracy or completeness of the contents of this book. The advice and strategies contained herein shall not be construed as medical, psychiatric or psychological treatment. You should consult with a professional where appropriate. Neither the publisher nor the author shall be held liable for any loss or damages.

ISBN-13:
978-1534669246

ISBN-10:
1534669248

Table of Contents

Introduction

The world we live in today is radically different than the one our grandparents grew up in. We have technology now that wasn't even dreamed of then. We have developed all kinds of products to make our lives better, or at least that is what they are supposed to do. Just think of the introduction of plastics. Look around you and see how many things are made of plastic. Our clothing and furniture contain synthetics. We are surrounded by things that didn't exist 100 years ago. Life changes at an ever increasing rate of speed and it is difficult to keep up with all the changes.

I want to say that I am pro-science. I have a background in life sciences and took the same science classes that pre-medical and pre-veterinary students take, prior to entry into my nursing and nurse practitioner programs. I don't think that "chemical" is a dirty word. I appreciate our advances in science. My concern is that we develop things, not looking so much at how they will benefit the human race and the planet, but based on the profit motive. As a result, we now have developed toxic substances and released them into the world without enough thought and testing about the safety and ethical use of these products.

I believe, as do many other scientists, that we are seeing ill effects on human health and on the environment as a result of short-sighted thinking that focuses on economics rather than the health of ourselves, our families and our world. Many studies on the safety of products are very brief and their long-term effects are unknown. They also look at one chemical at a time, one exposure to that chemical and don't consider the multiple chemicals we are being exposed to on a daily basis over a period of years. What could be safe if you just had one exposure to one chemical might not be safe when exposed multiple times to a mixture of chemicals that might interact with each other. The body is designed to cope with small exposures to toxins but can be overwhelmed when exposed to multiple toxins continuously. It is these multiple, continuous exposures that can increase our risk of disease. Our children are being exposed to toxins before they are even born and the longer we live, the more exposure we have had. It is time for us to take a step back, look at what is happening and take steps to protect ourselves.

Science is generally guided by the Precautionary Principle, which states:

"When an activity raises threats of harm to human health or the environment, precautionary measures should be taken even if some cause and effect relationships are not fully established scientifically" (Wingspread Conference on the Precautionary Principle". The Science and Environmental Health Network. January 26, 1998.).

This principle is followed more often in Europe than in the United States. There are many instances of it being completely ignored in the interest of profits. As a result, we are surrounded by known and suspected toxins.

But our government protects us, you say. Certainly they can't put things on the market that are dangerous, can they? I wish I could tell you that government agencies do rigorous testing on everything and don't approve things until they are proven to be safe. It is simply not the case. Most often, the company wanting to sell the product does some sort of testing that indicates the product is probably safe. These studies may be too short or even biased because the company wants the results to say their product is okay. They submit these studies to the government agencies.

There are all kinds of politics involved, not to mention the problem with money in politics, lobbying from industry and so forth. Many of the people running the government agencies that regulate various industries come from the industries they are supposed to regulate. This should certainly be seen as a conflict of interest but we continue to have a revolving door of people from industry working in regulatory agencies and then returning to the industry. I will briefly address some examples of this later and how it has affected our safety.

Another problem is that sometimes it takes years for the toxic effects to show up. If you are looking at whether a particular substance causes cancer, you might have to wait 20 years for it to show up in the increase in cancer rates. And even if you can show that people exposed to chemical X have a 25% greater chance of having cancer, does that prove that chemical X caused the cancer? Maybe the people who used the product with chemical X also used something else that was the actual causative agent. Can you see how difficult it could be to look at everything in a person's life to try to identify a causative agent? Think of how long it took to prove that smoking tobacco caused cancer. So sometimes we don't have definitive answers and need to use the precautionary principle if something might be a risk.

We know that there have been increases in conditions such as cancer and autism and there is a lot of finger pointing at particular potential causes such as GMOs and vaccines. I propose that it is probably not one thing but the combination of toxins in our environment interacting in our bodies. By reducing our overall toxic load, we decrease our risk of disease.

One of the things that really brought this to my attention and encouraged me to research the effects of toxins was an incident where I found some mold growing in my home. I used a commercial product designed to kill mold. I was unaware that some molds will produce mycotoxins, poisons that they release into the air, especially when attacked. I have a chronic disease called fibromyalgia and following the attack on the mold, I was sick for a month with what seemed to be an exacerbation or flare of the fibromyalgia but I could also feel a tightness in my lungs for several months. Since I normally keep my fibromyalgia fairly well controlled with diet and supplements so that I rarely have a flare (brief ones for a day or two), this was quite significant. The more I read about environmental toxins, the more I wanted to share what I was learning with others so that they could take action to reduce the toxins they were being exposed to.

The goal of this book is to help you make decisions about what products you eat, drink, purchase or allow in your home. Knowledge is power and if we quit buying toxic products, companies will quit making them and start making something non-toxic that will sell. You can see this in the growth of the organic food industry. We started buying organic food and the big companies, like PepsiCo, Coca-Cola, Kellogg's and General Mills , noticed and have bought a lot of the companies producing organic products because they want to get into that very lucrative market. Corporations are very aware of what sells. Every time we purchase something, we are voting with our dollars about what kind of products we want produced. Consumer knowledge and pressure is what is going to produce change and I want to give you the knowledge you need for a safer world for you, your children and grandchildren.

Chapter One

What Are You Eating?

The industrialization of agriculture has made it so that we eat less real, fresh food and more food-like products that are processed and contain preservatives, additives to enhance flavor and artificial colors to provide a more appealing color. Even the fresh food we eat may be laced with pesticides or other chemicals, not to mention that many foods are now genetically modified, a process that is not nearly as safe as the chemical companies that produce these foods would have you believe.

Let's start with GMOs (genetically modified organisms). The biotech/chemical companies that have created genetically modified foods would have you believe that this is a fairly straightforward process where they take a gene that codes for a trait that they want and put it into a cell. They also infer that what they do is not much different than the breeding of plants and animals that has been done for generations to create plants and animals with desirable traits.

In traditional methods, you are using the same or extremely similar organisms and breeding for an improved version of that organism. This is the process by which humans took animals that were basically tamer versions of wolves and turned them into basset hounds, Chihuahuas and Great Danes. It is how they bred white flowering plants with red flowering plants and got pink flowering plants. The difference here is that you are just creating genetic variations of the same species. You are not trying to mix petunias with giraffes.

Genetically modified organisms are created to do things that are quite different from what the original does. For example, BT corn actually produces an insecticide, BT toxin. When this insecticide is sprayed on a food, it breaks down with sunlight and washes off. When it is produced by the corn plant, it can't be washed off because it is inside the corn so that you are getting a dose of it when you eat the corn. BT toxin doesn't have an effect on humans but what about all those micro-organisms that live in your intestines? Those little guys are essential to your health. Just how important they are has been the focus of a lot of recent research. Did anyone consider that ingesting pesticides might not be good for them?

The most commonly known genetically modified foods are Round-Up Ready corn and soy. By Round-Up Ready, they mean that these corn and soy plants can be sprayed with Round-Up, an herbicide that normally kills plants, and will not be harmed by it. So the farmer can spray his field of Round-Up Ready crops with Round-Up and it will kill the weeds and leave his corn or soy untouched. Seems like a great idea, right? Except for the little problem of glyphosate, the active ingredient in Round-Up, being a probable carcinogen and also linked to liver and kidney damage.

Monsanto, the company that makes the Round-Up ready seeds and Round-Up was quite upset when the World Health Organization came out and called glyphosate a probable carcinogen. Not that it should have been a surprise to them since their own records show that they knew about this 35 years ago.

Much of this GMO corn and soy is used to feed animals and there have also been some animal studies that indicate that there may be a link to gastric inflammation, reduced fertility and an increase in fetal malformations. There is also the research done by Gilles-Eric Seralini, a professor at the University of Caen, France, on rats, showing that after a period of several months of eating GMOs, the rats began developing liver and kidney damage, pituitary gland damage and mammary gland tumors (the rat equivalent of breast cancer). This research was published by a peer-reviewed journal in 2012, then suddenly it was retracted. This was apparently due to pressure from biotech companies. It took several years of the research being reviewed before it was once again upheld as valid and made public.

There were no tests as to whether any of the GMO foods were safe for human consumption. How can this be, you ask? The United States government and most of the other governments in the world have a policy of promoting the biotech industry. So even if scientists at the FDA or USDA may question their safety, the political appointees that head these agencies have a different agenda. Unless, there is overwhelming, irrefutable evidence of immediate harm (which is almost impossible to prove), then no action will be taken. This is because Monsanto has claimed that their food is not different than the food already on the market so it is classified under the GRAS list. GRAS means "generally regarded as safe" and foods on this list require no testing at all. The recent head of the FDA, Michael Taylor, is largely responsible for this classification. He is a former attorney for Monsanto and has gone back and forth between working for the FDA and Monsanto.

These GMO seeds were different enough that Monsanto and other chemical companies were able to obtain patents but are considered the same as non-GMO foods when it comes to FDA or USDA regulations. As a result, you and I are guinea pigs for these new foods. GMOs are found in over 70% of the foods on your grocery store shelves.

Back in the 1980's, I got to know a woman who was in a wheelchair as a result of a condition called eosinophilia-myalgia syndrome. She got this as a result of taking contaminated tryptophan. Tryptophan is an amino acid that is found in our food and our bodies and many people were using it as a supplement. This particular batch of tryptophan tablets that were contaminated were traced back to one manufacturer in Japan. At the time, I thought that they must have accidentally added a contaminant somehow during processing. All tryptophan supplements were banned following the outbreak of this disorder.

It was only recently when researching GMOs that I discovered that the tryptophan involved was produced by genetically modified bacteria. There had been an attempt to determine how the contamination occurred. The processing that took place after the bacterial production of the tryptophan was examined closely but failed to find anything. By the time the investigation got around to looking at the genetically engineered bacteria themselves, they had all been destroyed. So, although it could not be proven, it appeared that the genetically modified bacteria were producing the contaminant along with the tryptophan. Genetically engineering bacteria is easier than modifying plants so if genetically modified bacteria have this kind of problem, the risk is even greater with more complex organisms such as plants or animals.

Genetic modification is a very complicated and difficult task. It is not the simple "take this gene and put it into that organism" process that biotech companies would have you believe. Finding the gene that is desired among all the DNA in an organism and then finding enzymes to cut that particular gene out is a daunting task but then you have to put it into the organism that you are trying to genetically modify. This is difficult with a simple one-celled bacteria but is infinitely more difficult when you are trying to put it into a complex organism like a plant or an animal. And there is no way to know what other genes might be turned on or off or what other effects could occur. And while all living organisms use DNA and RNA, there are incompatibilities between the DNA of bacteria and complex organisms. Even with modifying genes to overcome that issue, there can be all kinds of unintended effects. The entire process is unnatural and full of risks.

One of the results of our use of genetically modified food plants is that there has been an increase in the use of herbicides, particularly glyphosate or Round-Up but also others. Because we are using poisons to kill weeds, those weeds that are least sensitive to the herbicide are the ones that are most likely to survive and reproduce so that "superweeds" that are resistant to the weed killer develop. So as the weeds become harder to kill, more Round-Up is used. In addition, the main component of Agent Orange, 2,4,-D, is now being added to the chemicals used to kill these superweeds. Agent Orange was used in Vietnam as a defoliant during the Vietnam War and has resulted in a variety of negative health effects for Vietnam Veterans. Another older chemical being used is Dicamba. Both of these are even worse for the environment than glyphosate.

Another aspect of the use of chemicals in agriculture is how it affects the soil. We don't tend to think too much about the soil our food is grown in but it contains lots of microorganisms that are important for the health of the plants. Use of pesticides can alter what microorganisms are present and can affect the fertility of the soil. In addition, glyphosate binds with some minerals present in the soil so that you are getting food with reduced mineral content. Recently, I read that glyphosate is killing earthworms which might account for farmers using the chemical reporting that their soil becomes hard and more compact after its use.

Besides herbicides, industrial agriculture uses a lot of insecticides. One class of these, the neonicotinoids, has been linked to the drastic reduction in the numbers of honeybees and butterflies. These beneficial insects are necessary for the pollination of many plants and without them, many of our food crops would disappear.

Pesticides have been implicated in many environmental problems ever since Rachel Carson brought to light the problems with DDT in her book, *Silent Spring*. They end up in our water thru run-off. All of the streams in the U.S. contain some level of pesticide residue. Children have pesticides in their developing bodies before birth and the older we get the more pesticide residues we have in our bodily tissues.

Washing or peeling can remove some of the pesticide residue from foods but not all. Foods that are highest in pesticide residue include:

- Apples
- Celery
- Sweet Bell Peppers
- Peaches
- Strawberries
- Nectarines (imported)
- Grapes
- Spinach
- Lettuce
- Cucumbers
- Blueberries
- Potatoes

You will want to only purchase organic versions of these foods. You will also want to buy organic versions of foods that are genetically modified since GMOs are not labeled. These foods include:

- Corn
- Canola
- Cottonseed
- Mangos
- Soy
- Sugar unless it clearly states that it is cane sugar (sugar beets have been genetically modified).
- Yellow crookneck or zucchini squash

In addition, glyphosate is now being sprayed on some non-GMO crops just prior to harvest. It kills the plant but apparently this is actually beneficial for harvesting. This means that these non-GMO crops are getting doused with glyphosate:

- Barley
- Beans
- Oats
- Peas
- Wheat

So, if it is a grain or something that comes from a pod, it can be sprayed with glyphosate, giving us another group of foods that we will need to buy organically grown.

If you are not vegan, you are getting additional substances you probably don't want from meat, poultry, fish, dairy products and eggs. Just for starters, unless you are buying organic meat, that animal was almost certainly fed GMOs. Most of the GMO corn and soy is fed to animals. Most of us picture farm animals as wandering free in a pasture, eating grass or whatever. In actuality, most of them spend their lives in Confined Animal Feeding Operations or CAFOs. Many states are now passing laws referred to as Ag-Gag laws that forbid whistleblowers from filming or taking pictures of what happens there because they don't want you to know. They want you to keep picturing those animals in the pasture when they are actually crowded together, often inside a big building.

Cows tend to be outside in feed lots but chickens and hogs are indoors and usually caged. The extreme crowding is unnatural and sometimes leads to behavior problems and cages prevent them from injuring each other. Sometimes chickens have been "debeaked" where the end of the beak is cut off to prevent injury from pecking by other chickens.

The goal of CAFOs is to produce as much meat, eggs, milk, etc. as quickly and cheaply as possible. So the animals are considered to be commodities, not sentient creatures. They are given cheap feed (which can even contain animal by-products and fish meal) and any synthetic chemicals that will make them grow faster. Two things that do this are hormones and antibiotics. Antibiotics can also help prevent disease since stressed, crowded animals are at higher risk for getting sick. Did you know that more antibiotics are given to livestock than are used for humans? This is a big concern for healthcare providers because it increases the chance for development of antibiotic resistant bacteria.

Hormones used are mostly synthetic versions of estrogen. There is some concern that we are getting too much estrogen because we get it from our food and that this could be related to the younger age of puberty in girls and the increase in breast cancer. Another one that is often used in dairy cows is recombinant bovine growth hormone (rBGH). It increases the amount of milk the cow gives and there are concerns about whether this could also be linked to the increase in breast cancer.

These CAFOs produce a lot of waste products. You can imagine the amount of urine and feces produced by thousands of animals crowded together. This can result in contamination of ground water or streams near these large enterprises. When animals are raised on pasture, the waste products become fertilizer but when the amount of waste produced far exceeds nature' ability to break it down and absorb it, it becomes a problem.

So, if you eat animal products, what can you do? If you have local farmers and farmer's markets in your community, you have an opportunity to talk to them about how they raise their animals and what they feed them. I've toured the local farm that sells the grass-fed beef that I buy and talked with the owner. If you don't have that option, look for labels that say 100% grass-fed and/or organic. If a product is organic, that means no GMOs, antibiotics or hormones have been used. If you see a label that says "natural", you need to be aware that this word generally means nothing. They are trying to con you into believing they didn't use anything artificial when they probably did.

You have probably seen "cage free" eggs. This does not mean that they hens have access to outdoors; it just means the owner took out the cages and let the hens loose in the warehouse. When eggs are certified organic, it means that the hens were not given anything artificial or genetically modified and that they have some access to outdoors. Ideally, you want eggs that are organic and "pastured", meaning that they spend a significant part of their time outdoors pecking and scratching the ground as hens are supposed to do. The yolks of these eggs are a yellowish orange instead of the pale yellow of commercial eggs. If you have room in your backyard and there are no ordinances against it, you might like to have a few chickens of your own. Not only will you get fresh eggs but they can be quite entertaining. You do not need roosters unless you want to have chicks.

You may have heard that pregnant women should not eat much tuna because it contains mercury. So even though fish are considered "healthy", we have to think about what kind of fish and where they came from. In general, larger fish that are eating smaller fish tend to accumulate more toxins because they ingest whatever toxins the small fish might have. Farmed fish are higher in toxins because of the way they are raised. Many fish species are being over fished. There are lots of considerations. The Environmental Working Group's suggestions for best choices are wild salmon, sardines, mussels, rainbow trout and atlantic mackerel. These are high in Omega-3 fatty acids and low in mercury.

You may wonder why fresh, healthy (organic) food is more expensive than foods that are high in grains and sugars. The highly processed junk food is made from crops that are subsidized by the government. That is correct. Farmers growing corn and soybeans get subsidies. The guy selling organic vegetables at the farmer's market has to pay extra to get his organic certification. None of this makes sense from a health perspective. It only makes sense when you follow the money. The large industrial farms form associations that hire lobbyists and get their people hired by government regulatory agencies so that they get benefits.

If you want healthy food for yourself and your family, opt out of the agribusiness produced food system. When you spend your money to buy organic, you are encouraging the growth of organic and sustainable farming in addition to reducing your intake of unwanted chemicals.

You can also grow your own so that you know exactly what you are getting and have the pleasure of harvesting things you have produced. Gardening is good exercise and is also good for your mental health. If you don't have land, do you have an area such as a patio where you can grow things in pots? What about a community garden?

If you aren't able to grow your own food, you might want to consider a CSA (community supported agriculture). Many small farms have a CSA program where you can purchase a "share" of what the farm produces. You pay the farmer up-front and then receive a box of whatever the farm is producing each week. Small families of one or two people can usually buy a half share.

A word of caution needs to be included about food you purchase. Even health food stores and alternative grocery stores can contain "junk food". You have to learn to read labels. Forget the nutritional label and go right for the list of ingredients. Foods are required to list ingredients according to the amount of each by weight. Many times manufacturers will attempt to confuse you by using different words to hide ingredients that people are familiar with and don't want. For example, if they don't want sugar as the first ingredient, they can put in smaller amounts of different sugars (if it ends in –ose, it is probably sugar). They know people are avoiding things like MSG and high fructose corn syrup so they may call them by different names.

It does not appear that we are going to get mandatory GMO labeling in the U.S. at this time, even though 90% of the population support labeling. Other countries that do have it, may lose it due to "free-trade" agreements. GMO labeling could be banned thru the use of lawsuits as a "barrier to trade" if "free-trade" agreements are implemented. We have already seen something similar happen under NAFTA (the North American Free Trade

Agreement) where there was a lawsuit from another country regarding the U.S. law requiring meat to be labeled with the country of origin. The U.S. Congress rescinded this law because of the lawsuit. So, we cannot trust that we will have GMO labeling and will have to learn to identify them on our own.

Just to start with, here is a list of ingredients which you may find in foods that, unless the product is certified organic or non-GMO, are probably GMO:

- aspartame
- baking powder
- canola oil
- caramel color
- cellulose
- citric acid
- cobalamin (vitamin B 12)
- condensed milk
- confectioners' sugar
- corn flour
- corn masa
- corn meal
- corn oil
- corn sugar
- corn syrup
- cornstarch
- cotton seed oil
- cyclodextrin
- cysteine
- dextrin
- dextrose
- diacetyl

19

- diglyceride
- erythritol
- Equal
- food starch
- fructose
- glucose
- glutamate
- glutamic acid
- glycerides
- glycerin
- glycerol
- glycerol monooleate
- glycine
- hemicellulose
- high fructose corn syrup (HFCS)
- hydrogenated starch
- hydrolyzed vegetable protein
- inositol
- inverse syrup
- inversol
- invert sugar
- isoflavones
- lactic acid
- lecithin
- leucine
- lysine
- malitol
- malt
- malt syrup
- malt extract,
- maltodextrin
- maltose,

- mannitol
- methylcellulose
- milk powder
- milo starch
- modified food starch
- modified starch
- mono and diglycerides
- monosodium glutamate (MSG)
- NutraSweet
- oleic acid
- phenylalanine
- phytic acid
- protein isolate
- sorbitol
- soy flour
- soy isolates
- soy lecithin
- soy milk
- soy oil
- soy protein
- soy protein isolate
- soy sauce
- starch
- stearic acid
- sugar (unless it specifically states that it is cane sugar)
- tamari
- tempeh
- teriyaki marinades
- textured vegetable protein
- threonine
- tocopherols (vitamin E)
- tofu

- triglyceride
- vegetable fat
- vegetable oil
- whey
- whey powder
- xanthan gum

You will notice some artificial sweeteners in that list. Even if these were not GMO, there are definite questions about their safety and they do not aid significantly in weight loss. In fact, diet soda has been linked to an increase in the incidence of diabetes and obesity. Artificial sweeteners are best avoided.

Sugar is inflammatory and should be used in moderation. It also promotes the growth of cancer. Our current intake of sugars is a far cry from moderation. Our intake of sugar increased steadily from 6.3 pounds per person per year in 1822 to a maximum of 107.7 pounds/person/year in 1999. That is 17 times as much. A lot of this is high fructose corn syrup which is suspected of having a much worse effect than sugar.

Sweetened drinks are particularly risky as a 12 ounce can of soda contains about 10 teaspoons of sugar (usually as high fructose corn syrup) and if you think that is bad, 12 ounces of orange juice has 12 teaspoons. Think agave nectar is better? Wrong. It is higher in fructose and processed so if you are trying to avoid obesity and diabetes, it is actually worse. For your health, you want to limit yourself to only occasional use of cane sugar, honey or maple syrup. Other sweeteners include Stevia (not the highly processed versions such as Truvia which also contains GMO erythritol) or certified non-GMO xylitol (not well digested so large amounts can cause diarrhea but doesn't have an aftertaste and can be used in cooking).

Another category of ingredient that you will want to use caution with are preservatives. These extend shelf life of processed foods. People have used methods to preserve food for millennia. Some of the common ways are to use things like salt, sugar (low levels encourage bacterial growth but very high levels inhibit it such as in making jam), pickling, drying, smoking and freezing. Ascorbic acid (also known as vitamin C) is a safe preservative. If you are eating fresh foods, you will not have to worry about these.

Nitrates and nitrites are found in processed meats such as bacon, hot dogs, lunch meat, ham and pastrami. That bright pink color in meat is a red flag. These are linked to cancer and lower life expectancy. It is possible to buy uncured meats without them; one must just be sure to keep them refrigerated and use them promptly.

BHA and BHT are derived from petroleum and used to preserve fats and oils. They are banned in many other countries but still used in the U.S. They have produced cancer in rats and mice.

Propyl gallate is used to keep oils fresh and is a central nervous system depressant that can cause kidney damage. It has also been linked to cancer in rats and may be an endocrine disruptor.

Sulfites are preservatives are often found in wine, dried fruit and prepared potatoes and are used to stop the discoloration of food, but have been linked to an asthma-related sensitivity and allergy in some cases.

Sodium benzoate is a preservative that helps stop the fermentation or acidification of foods. It can be found in sodas and fruit juices. It is possible that when sodium benzoate is mixed with ascorbic acid, it could create benzene, a carcinogen.

TBHQ (Tert-ButylHydroQuinone) is a synthetic antioxidant preservative similar to BHA. It increased the incidence of tumors in rats.

Some other things you may find in your food include thickening agents, coloring agents and antifoaming agents. Here are a few of them.

Carrageenan is an indigestible, thickening agent that comes from seaweed. There are some concerns about its effects on the colon, particularly in infants (it can be found in infant formula). It is probably not good for people with gastrointestinal problems and some people have found relief from gastrointestinal distress with its elimination. While it is could be a problem in large quantities, most people are okay with the small amounts in food.

Caramel coloring is often found in bread (to make it look like whole wheat) and in sodas plus many other foods. It is one of the most common food additives. It is produced by heating sugar but has ammonia compounds added in processing. In 2011, the International Agency for Research on Cancer, a division of the World Health Organization, concluded that some of the compounds that are found in caramel coloring are "possibly carcinogenic to humans."

Potassium bromate and azodicarbonamide (ADC) are both additives to bread flour that have been linked to cancer.

Propyl paraben, a thickening agent, is an endocrine disrupting chemical that can decrease sperm counts.

Dimethylpolysiloxane is an antifoaming agent similar to silicone found in some fast foods (and cosmetics). When you see things on labels that you can't pronounce and don't understand, it is probably best to research them or avoid them.

Then we have artificial food colors. The Center on Science in the Public Interest (CSPI) summarizes their research on food colors as follows: *"The three most widely used dyes, Red 40, Yellow 5, and Yellow 6, are contaminated with known carcinogens ... Another dye, Red 3, has been acknowledged for years by the Food and Drug Administration to be a carcinogen, yet is still in the food supply."* For more information, you might want to read their 58 page report, "Food Dyes: a rainbow of risks".

Companies use artificial colors because they are cheap and make the food appear more attractive. If we quit buying their brightly colored artificial food, they will start producing more natural products. Once again, it is up to you to think about what is in your food and vote with your purchasing behavior for the kind of food you want.

If you have been eating food with high levels of pesticides or if you have taken antibiotics, it is helpful to replace the good bacteria that have been killed with the use of probiotics or fermented food such as homemade sauerkraut, kimchi, kombucha, kefir or yogurt. The commercial versions have been pasteurized so you want to make these yourself to get the beneficial micro-organisms. You can find recipes and instructions for doing this online. If you are taking probiotics, get a good one that requires refrigeration and has a lot of micro-organisms in it, not just lactobacillus. These can be pricey but you get what you pay for. Cheap ones won't work as well.

You may have heard about a condition referred to as "leaky gut" which has been linked to a number of chronic diseases including auto-immune diseases. Research on this is new and not widely accepted by the medical community yet but this is a result of disruption of the "microbiome", as the ecological system of micro-organisms in your body is referred to. Your goal is to increase the number of healthy microbes (and those help keep the disease-causing ones in control).

In summary,

- Find sources for fresh, local, healthy food. Know your farmer. Consider gardening, if you aren't already doing it, or join a CSA
- Learn to read ingredient labels so you know what is in any food that has a combination of ingredients.
- Know which foods are genetically modified and which are high in pesticides so that you can buy organic versions of those foods.
- Support the healthy bacteria in your gut by taking a probiotic or eating naturally fermented (not pasteurized) foods.

Chapter Two
What's in your Water?

Water is a critical nutrient for health so having clean, non-toxic drinking water is important. Drinking coffee, tea, soda or energy drinks with caffeine can actually increase your need for water since these are diuretics. Drinking soda or other sugary liquids is also detrimental to health so learning to drink water instead is a very good habit. If you live somewhere that has poor quality water with an objectionable taste, this can be a problem.

Many people now choose to drink bottled water, thinking that this is better for them than tap water. In some areas, the taste is certainly better but as far as health is concerned, bottled water may actually be worse than what is coming out of your tap. In many cases, bottled water may actually be tap water however you are adding the risk of chemicals such as BPA (Bisphenol-A) from the plastic getting into your water, especially if it is exposed to sunlight. BPA is a hormone disrupting chemical that has been in the news a lot so that you may see "BPA free" on some plastic containers now. Usually, they are simply switching to another chemical that is not significantly better. We will discuss it more in the next chapters on plastics. You are much better off getting a stainless steel water bottle to carry water with you.

In a recent German study, 24,500 chemicals were found in bottled water. This included two classes of drugs, maleates and fumarates that are used to make plastic resins and water bottles. These are known endocrine disruptors and the study found that estrogenic activity was inhibited by 60 percent and androgenic activity by 90 percent. Tap water, on the other hand, did not affect estrogen or androgen receptors. This is especially important for small children and pregnant women but others should also avoid these since they can increase the risk of diabetes, heart disease and even cancer.

There are legally enforceable standards for drinking water which state what maximum levels of contaminants are okay in drinking water. For some of these, particularly micro-organisms, the level is zero. The other types of contaminants include disinfectants such as chlorine that is added to water to kill microorganisms, disinfection byproducts, inorganic chemicals and organic chemicals.

Some chemicals that we need to be concerned about include the following:

- Antimony: This can affect cholesterol and blood sugar and comes from petroleum refineries, fire retardants and electronics.
- Arsenic: This is a carcinogenic substance that can get into the water thru runoff from natural deposits as well as industrial wastes.
- Asbestos: It can cause intestinal polyps and can come from cement and natural deposits
- Aluminum: It competes with calcium for skeletal absorption and interferes with the absorption of phosphorus, zinc and selenium.
- Chlorine: This is added to the city water supplies to sterilize them so is necessary but should be filtered out as it can destroy beneficial microorganisms in

the body. One of the breakdown products of chlorine is chloroform gas which increases the risk of airway irritation and asthma, dizziness, nausea and fatigue.

- Fluoride: This has been deliberately added to our water as it is supposed to prevent tooth decay. More recent studies have cast doubt on this and other studies have shown it to be neurotoxic resulting in lower IQs in children who are exposed to it. In addition, it is an endocrine disruptor. In particular, it adversely affects the thyroid. The form of fluoride added to our water is actually an industrial waste product. It is corrosive and has a detrimental effect on lead pipes so could also increase the risk of lead in your water. Many municipalities are now taking a second look and deciding to stop adding it to their water supplies. If your community fluoridates their water, you might want to find others who are concerned and see if you can get your city to stop this practice.
- Lead: This can get into the water from corroded pipes and is linked to learning disorders and developmental delays.

Some other things that can get into the water include disinfectant byproducts such as trihalomethane and halogenic acetic acid which are used along with chlorine to disinfect water. These can cause cancer, liver and kidney disease and affect the nervous system. It is also possible for small amounts of prescription and over-the-counter drugs to end up in the water supply. There are also estrogenic chemicals and some that are anti-androgenic which can lead to feminizing effects such as gynecomastia, otherwise known as "man boobs".

If you have not had your water tested, I would recommend that you do so. That will let you know what chemicals you may be dealing with. You should also consider what sort of filtering you want to use. For most people a simple carbon filter is adequate for removing contaminants and improving taste but if you have fluoridated water, a carbon filter will not eliminate fluoride and you will want to install a reverse osmosis system. A system for the entire house is expensive but many people have a smaller system for their kitchen so that they have clean water for drinking and cooking. If fluoride isn't an issue, you can get pitchers that filter water which are quite inexpensive. You can also get a carbon filter for your shower.

Since the city closest to me has fluoridated water, I chose to buy a home outside the city with a well and had the water tested before moving in. I have a water pitcher with a filter in my refrigerator so that I always have access to plenty of good tasting, clean water.

In summary:
- Water is important for health and is better than sodas and other drinks.
- Avoid bottled water. Get a stainless steel water bottle that you can fill with filtered tap water to take with you.
- Have your tap water tested.
- Decide what system of filtering is best for you and use it.

Chapter Three

Cleanliness Can Be Dangerous

Our culture has become obsessed with cleanliness and killing germs. This is no surprise as we are bombarded with advertisements for disinfecting this and antibacterial that. What these advertisements never tell you is that your body is host to around 100 trillion microbes (bacteria, viruses and funguses). You have about 10 times more microorganisms than you do human cells. The largest amount of these are the ones that live in your gut but you also have a lot on the skin and other areas of your body.

We have always had these microbes and without them we would die. They are vital for health, for nutrition, for immunity to disease and for effects on your brain and behavior. The ones that live in your gut weigh about four pounds; considering how tiny they are, that's a lot of microbes! There are pathogenic microbes that can cause disease but usually these are kept in check by the beneficial ones. Microbes play a variety of roles and disturbances in the balance of microbes has been implicated in many diseases including allergies, asthma, autism, autoimmune conditions, cancer, diabetes, eczema, heart disease, intestinal problems such as celiac disease, colitis and irritable bowel syndrome, multiple sclerosis and obesity. Without exposure to microorganisms, we would not develop the part of our immune system that responds quickly to microbes that cause disease. This starts at birth with exposure to vaginal microbes during travel down the birth canal. There has actually been research recently that

34

shows that children who play in the dirt, who have dogs who go outside and bring in germs from outside or who live on farms tend to be healthier.

So now we know that we can relax about killing germs, we don't need to buy products with chlorine bleach, Triclosan (an insecticide found in most antibacterial soaps) or other sanitizing products. Simply washing with soap and warm water and drying with a clean towel works just fine. Proper handwashing is better than hand sanitizer for removing excess germs. Sponges, dishcloths, dish towels and cutting boards can harbor bacteria. If you are going to use sponges, run them through the dishwasher. Otherwise, switch to dishcloths that you can wash frequently. Dish towels also need to be washed frequently. Wood cutting boards are less likely to harbor germs but it is a good idea to have a separate one for meat and always wash cutting boards with soap and water after using.

Besides those antibacterial and antiviral ingredients, cleaning agents and cosmetics contain plenty of other toxins that you will also want to avoid. The United States government currently does very little to regulate chemicals in cosmetics, personal care products or cleaning products. In fact, the FDA actually states that they do not have the legal authority to approve cosmetics before they go on the market. The chemical industry has a strong lobby in Washington so it is very hard to get effective regulations. The European Union bans over 1100 chemicals that are found in U.S. products. This allows you to inhale or absorb through your skin, a variety of toxic chemicals.

Let's start with cosmetics and personal care products since we actually apply these directly to the skin to not only clean, but to make ourselves more attractive and, in some cases, to try to prevent aging. This means you have prolonged contact with these ingredients so that they can absorb through your skin. Manufacturers can pretty much use any substances and make any claims they want. Unless the product causes actual damage such as the "Brazilian" formaldehyde hair straighteners that the FDA investigated in 2010 after receiving reports of hair damage and scalp burns, no action is generally taken. In the case of the hair straightening products, the agency sent a warning letter but didn't remove the products from the market.

So what are some ingredients that you will want to avoid? Here is a list:

- **BHA** and **BHT** are used in make-up and in moisturizers as preservatives. We discussed these in the chapter on food. These are suspected endocrine disruptors and BHA has been linked to cancer.
- **Coal tar/ dyes/coloring agents** can also be called p-phenylenediamine hair dyes or FD&C Blue #1, FD&C Red #6 and so forth. They have the potential to cause cancer and are often contaminated with heavy metals
- **DEA** and related ingredients, **MEA** and **TEA**, are used in foaming or creamy products. They can react to form nitrosamines which are carcinogenic.
- **Formaldehyde releasing products** include **DMDM hydantion, diazolidinyl urea, imidazolidinyl urea, methenamine and quarternium-15.** These can be

found in water-based cosmetics, deodorants, hair dyes, shaving creams and face masks. They work in conjunction with parabens as preservatives. Formaldehyde is a carcinogen.

- **Fragrance** is a vague term that can include a variety of things but one of them is generally phthalates (see below). Fragrances can cause headaches, dizziness, asthma and allergies.
- **Heavy Metals** are not deliberately added but are common contaminants found in cosmetics. These include arsenic, beryllium, cadmium, lead, selenium and thallium. Lip gloss and lipstick are especially risky products that may contain arsenic, cadmium and lead. Since you are applying these to your mouth, you are ingesting them orally. The tiny amounts found in cosmetic products wouldn't be a concern with a single use but since these substances accumulate in the body, years of exposure could lead to health problems.
- **Hydroquinone** is used for lightening skin. It is linked to cancer and reproductive toxicity and is banned in the UK.
- **Parabens** is used as an anti-microbial preservative. It may be listed as **methylparabens, propylparabens** or **butyl parabens** and is an endocrine disruptor.
- **PEG compounds** such as **polyethylene glycol** can be contaminated with 1,4-dioxane, a carcinogen. **Propylene glycol** is a related chemical.
- **Petroleum products** such as **mineral oil** are used because they are cheap and can provide shine or a moisture barrier. They are not good for your skin and can be contaminated with polycyclic aromatic hydrorcarbons, which may cause cancer.

- **Phthalates** are used in the manufacturing of plastic to make it soft and flexible but are also found in plastic wrap, lubricants, detergents, insecticides and in your cosmetics. They are often found in products with fragrance to stabilize it so if the label has fragrance, you can bet it has phthalates too. Phthalates are endocrine disruptors and contribute to early onset of puberty. They may be listed as **dibutylphthalate (DBP), dimethylphthalate (DMP), or diethylphthalate (DEP)**.
- **PVP/VA copolymer** is used as a binder or fixer in cosmetics but is a respiratory and skin irritant.
- **Retinyl palmitate** is a vitamin A derivative that may be found in sunscreens and anti-aging products. In a study of mice, application of retinyl palmitate and exposure to sunlight caused tumors.
- **Silicone derivatives** are not biodegradable and irritate the skin. They have been linked to the growth of tumors.
- **Sodium lauryl sulfate** is the stuff that makes soaps, shampoos and cleansers foamy. It is absorbed into your body and irritates the skin.
- **Stearalkonium Chloride** is found in hair conditioner and creams to prevent static and hair frizzing and as a preservative. It is an allergen and a suspected environmental toxin.
- **Talc** has been linked to ovarian cancer. This is found in baby powder, deodorant, eye shadow, blush and face powder.
- **Toluene** is found in nail and hair products and is an endocrine disruptor that can affect the immune system and fetal development.

- **Triclosan** is a common ingredient in antibacterial soaps, hand sanitizers, deodorants and toothpaste. It is linked to cancer and is an endocrine disruptor.
- **Triethanolamine** is used to balance pH in lotions and mascara. It is a skin and respiratory irritant, is toxic to the immune system and has been linked to cancer in laboratory animals.

This is quite a list and you will find it a challenge to find products which do not contain any of these ingredients from most retailers. There are two ways to get better cosmetics and personal care products. The first is to make your own and you can find some recipes on the internet. Since safe cosmetics tend to be more expensive, this is a good way to save money and know exactly what is in your products. If you don't want to go to the effort of buying ingredients and making your own, you can use the Environmental Working Group's Skin Deep online database which rates different products so you can see which ones are the safest.

Another consideration is whether your products are tested on animals. As an animal advocate and a supporter of the Beagle Freedom Project, a group which rescues beagles and other animals from labs where they have been used for testing, I don't want to use products that are tested on animals. There are ways to use cell cultures rather than animals. These animals (often beagles but sometimes other dogs, pigs, rabbits and cats) live their entire lives in cages where they are subjected to tests which are often painful and when the testing is over, are usually killed. The Beagle Freedom Project works with labs to take these animals and place them in homes instead of being killed. They have an app for your cell phone which will allow you to see which products have been tested on animals: cruelty-cutter.org

If you think the ingredients in personal care and cosmetic products are bad, those in cleaning products for your house are worse. They are also unregulated with the exception of the EPA requiring products with antibacterial agents to identify them. If you are reading labels and ingredients lists, you may have noticed that it is difficult to figure out what a product contains due to incomplete labeling. Once again the Environmental Working Group (ewg.org) rates products to find the safest ones. Some products should be avoided completely. These include air fresheners, fabric softeners, caustic drain cleaners and oven cleaners.

Many cleaning products are harmful to the lungs and can trigger asthma. Some use formaldehyde, a human carcinogen, as a preservative. Chlorinated phenols found in toilet bowl cleaners are toxic to the respiratory and circulatory systems. All purpose and windows cleaners may contain diethylene glycol, a nervous system depressant, nonylphenol ethoxylate, which has been banned in Europe due to toxicity, and butyl cellosolve which damages the bone marrow, kidneys, liver and nervous system. Floor cleaners can contain petroleum solvents that damage mucous membranes. Spot cleaners may contain perchloroethylene which causes liver and kidney damage. You get the idea. Even borax also known as sodium borate or boric acid, which I thought was fairly safe, turns out to be an endocrine disruptor.

There are "green" products available but even then you want to check because some of these products claiming to be "safe" or non-toxic might not be. An example is Simple Green Concentrated All-Purpose Cleaner. It says it is non-toxic but it contains 2-butoxyethanol, a solvent that is absorbed through the skin which damages red blood cells and irritates the eyes.

Want to save money and be sure that your cleaning agent is non-toxic? Buy yourself a gallon of white vinegar, a big box of baking soda and a few spray bottles. Fill a spray bottle with half water and half vinegar and you have an all-purpose cleaner for countertops, windows, sinks and appliances. If you want a scented version, you can add several drops of an essential oil of your choice. Vinegar has disinfecting properties and is good for removing soap scum and hard water deposits. It also can be used straight for treating mold (wash it off with soap and water then spray the area with vinegar and let dry) and for killing weeds (spray on leaves; it may take several applications but it sure beats toxic products like Round-Up).

If you want to clean your oven or scour your stainless steel sink, spray with the vinegar water and then sprinkle some baking soda or Bar Keepers Friend to make a paste for scrubbing. The combination of vinegar water and baking soda works for toilets too. You can help keep your drains clean by putting some baking soda over the drain and pouring straight vinegar on it to create a foaming cleaner.

To make a wood cleaner/dusting spray, mix water with equal amounts of Murphy's Oil Soap. You can add essential oils for fragrance if desired. Spray lightly and wipe off with a soft cloth. This works on wood floors too.

I don't know about you, but I don't even like to walk down the aisle where the laundry products are in a grocery store. The overwhelming fragrance in the air makes me want to gag. Anne Steinemann, a professor at the University of Washington did a study of top-selling laundry products and air fresheners and found that they gave off almost 100 volatile organic compounds which were not listed on the labels and that five of the six products tested emitted one or more carcinogenic, hazardous air pollutants. Two national surveys found that 20 percent of the population reported adverse health effects from air fresheners and about 10 percent had adverse effects from laundry products. Among those who had asthma, the complaints were twice as high. Many laundry detergents now offer a "free and clear" version to avoid some of the fragrances that trigger allergies and asthma.

I quit using fabric softeners or dryer sheets years ago and have not missed them. IF you have hard water, you might want to put a little vinegar in your rinse cycle. If you really want to make your laundry smell good (and save on your utility bill), put up a clothesline. This is especially good for drying sheets and pillowcases.

There are green laundry detergents which will help you avoid other toxins besides just the fragrances. Some of the highly rated products from the Environmental Working Group include Seventh Generation Natural Powder Laundry Detergent, Dr. Bronner's 18-in-1 Hemp Pure Castile Soaps (I use these, diluted with water, for hand soap and body wash), Biokleen Laundry Liquid or Powder, and Planet 2x Ultra Laundry Liquid.

If you have a dishwasher, Seventh Generation, Biokleen, Earth Friendly, Sun and Earth, Green Shield Organic and Honest Co. are some good brands. If you hand wash your dishes, some good brands are Biokleen, BabyGanics, Planet, Grab Green, Better Life Dish It Out, Sun and Earth, Puracy and AspenClean. If you haven't already done so, you probably want to put the www.ewg.org website in your favorites or bookmarked sites so you can refer to it whenever you want to check out a product or get recommendations.

I mentioned air fresheners as products you don't want to use. This includes sprays, plug-ins, solid or liquid products, scented candles and scented wax melts. What can you use instead? If you have a wax melt warmer, you can use some coconut oil and essential oils in it. Essential oils can also be used in diffusers or you can mix them with water in a spray bottle.

There is no way to avoid exposure to all toxic cleaning products, soaps and fragrances but at least you can control the products used in your home to reduce your exposure significantly.

In Summary:
- Avoid antibacterial products.
- Learn to use the www.ewg.org website to check out cosmetics, personal care products, cleaning products and other household products containing chemicals to find the least toxic ones.
- Avoid products with fragrance. Substitute essential oils for artificial fragrances.
- Consider making your own products using simple, non-toxic ingredients.

Chapter Four

What's in Your House?

While we are frequently replacing food, cosmetics and cleaning products, items such as furniture last for many years. Some people have symptoms that make it worthwhile to replace items that are making them sick. But often they are unaware of what might be causing those symptoms. For all of us, it is good to be aware of possible toxins in our homes.

Let's start with upholstered furniture like sofas. If your sofa was manufactured before 2013, it probably contains flame retardants. 85% of sofa cushions contain toxic or untested flame retardants according to researchers from Duke University and UC Berkeley. 41% of them contained cholorinated Tris, a carcinogen that was banned for use in baby pajamas in the 1970's. Polybrominated diphenyl ethers (PBDE) are flame retardants that leach out of foam and fabric. Studies show that these chemicals can cause thyroid and neurobehavioral problems in newborn animals. The effect on humans is unknown but they should be considered toxins. Another flame retardant, Firemaster 550 is found more in newer sofas and is an endocrine disruptor in animals. Its health effects on humans are unknown. These chemicals don't stay in the furniture but are found in house dust, often at higher levels than the federal health guidelines recommend.

Mattresses are another item that can contain flame retardants. In addition, they, and your upholstered furniture, can contain:

46

- **Polyurethane foam**, which is a petroleum material that emits volatile organic compounds (VOCs). These VOCs are what causes a chemical odor. Polyurethane foam contains chemical catalysts, surfactants, emulsifiers and pigments which can cause possible cardiac arrhythmias, breathlessness, chest discomfort, irritation of mucous membranes, headache, coughing, dizziness, fatigue and blurred vision.
- **Rebonded foam** is a multi-colored pressed type of foam made of shredded leftovers which are bound together using a glue or adhesive. The adhesives may also give off VOCs and this foam is usually less durable than new foam. It is also found in carpet pads.
- **Adhesives** used to bond mattress layers can contain hazardous chemicals such as acetone, benzene, formaldehyde, ethylene chloride and other VOCs.
- **Cotton** is used on the inside and in the cover of mattresses. Organic cotton is a good choice but regular cotton is sprayed heavily with pesticides then treated with bleach and other additives.
- **Wool** is used in some more expensive mattresses and is less flammable than other products. Unless it is organic, it may be treated with pesticides and chemicals.
- **Polyester** is often used as a filling in mattresses and pillows as well as part of the covering fabric. Polyester is a petroleum product and can contain chemical residues. It is highly flammable and not environmentally friendly.
- **Memory foam** is a type of polyurethane foam made of petroleum polymers but contains some

toxic chemicals that are of special concern. These include **methylene dianiline** (MDA) which is a suspected carcinogen that causes eye and skin irritation, **vinilideine chloride**, another suspected carcinogen that causes eye and respiratory irritation, **methylbenzene or toluene** which can affect the nervous system, **dimethyformamide** which can possibly cause organ damage and cancer and **acetone** which is toxic in large amounts. Many people have reported sensitivity to memory foam mattresses.

- **Latex** can be either natural latex, made from the sap of rubber trees or synthetic latex made of styrene-butadiene rubber. Styrene is toxic, and possibly carcinogenic. Butadiene is a known carcinogen, a suspected teratogen and a mucous membrane irritant. Sometimes latex is blended with polyurethane or natural and synthetic latex are blended with each other. Blended latex can be called natural latex if it contains at least 30% natural latex.

- **Springs or coils** can act as an incubator for dust mites, mold and mildew because these provide a dark, damp area.

Considering that we spend about one-third of our life in our beds, getting a good mattress with as few toxins or irritants as possible is a wise choice. Organic mattresses made of natural products are available but are expensive. If you don't want to replace your mattress right now, a less costly method is to wrap your mattress completely with a polyethylene sheet that is at least 5 mils thick, then get an organic cotton cover.

Next, let's consider solid furniture. The best choices are solid wood, metal and glass. Much of the "wood" furniture produced today is made with manufactured wood products like particleboard, fiberboard and plywood which probably contain urea-formaldehyde glues. Even real wood can have stains and finishes containing benzene, toluene and methylene chloride. These toxins are given off as gasses for about five years. If you have furniture over five years old that hasn't been refinished or reupholstered, you are probably okay.

If you are buying new furniture, look for wood furniture made out of FSC certified wood and low or no VOC stains and finishes. Look for upholstered furniture with sustainable fabrics that are not stain resistant and with natural latex cushions.

Flooring is another source of VOCs. Of the 400 compounds that have been identified as VOCs in the home, 200 of them are found in carpets. Synthetic carpeting is made from plastic fibers from petroleum and is usually installed using solvent based adhesives. These emit toxic gases and can cause headaches, asthma, allergic reactions and dizziness. Natural fibers such as wool, cotton, sisal or jute and solvent-free adhesives can be used instead.

I prefer hard flooring such as wood or tile because it is easier to keep clean. Pressure treated wood is preferable to wood that has been treated with preservatives and phenol resins emit fewer toxins than urea resins. If you finish your floors with polyurethane, you will want to stay somewhere else for a week and keep the windows open. Using linseed oil is a safer alternative. Bamboo is a good, sustainable type of flooring but you will want to get FSC certified bamboo flooring that is formaldehyde free because the resin normally used has formaldehyde. Laminates can contain a variety of chemicals and resins.

Vinyl flooring contains PVC (polyvinyl chloride) which can cause cancer, birth defects, chronic bronchitis, skin diseases and liver dysfunction among other things. It also contains phthalates. If it is over five years old, it has probably off gassed the dangerous fumes. If you are considering new flooring, think about ceramic or terra cotta tile or a natural linoleum made from linseed oil.

PVC is found in many home products. You are probably not going to want to tear out your plumbing system to replace the PVC pipes but you can make sure that your shower curtain, anything with artificial leather or a plastic covering, plastic furniture and plastic tablecloths do not contain it. We will talk more about it under plastics.

You might want to choose a different window covering than mini blinds made of PVC. Sunlight makes them break down faster. Heavy metals may be used to stabilize the PVC and older ones can also give off lead dust as they deteriorate. Better choices include wood or bamboo blinds or washable curtains.

You have no doubt noticed that formaldehyde is mentioned frequently. This seems surprising since it is classified as a carcinogen by the International Agency for

Research on Cancer and a probable human carcinogen by the CDC. Some people are more sensitive to it than others and it can cause watery eyes, burning sensation, nausea and difficulty breathing. It can also cause people to become allergic to other chemicals. Things that will help include keeping the temperature low since heat makes it volatize more easily. Another thing you can do with things like pressed wood furniture and cabinets is to apply a product such as AFM Safe Seal, a water-based, low gloss sealer for porous surfaces.

Paints and craft supplies are another possible source of toxins. Latex paints are preferable to oil based ones and it is possible to purchase no or low VOC paints. Stains, thinners and paint strippers also contain dangerous toxins such as benzene, toluene, xylene and methylene chloride. If you need a solvent use a non-chlorinated one such as turpentine, ethanol or acetone. When using any of these products be sure to have good ventilation. Avoid spray paints since this will lead to even more inhalation of fumes. If you enjoy arts and crafts, be sure to read labels. Follow directions and heed the warnings on the package. Dry erase markers are one of the worst since they contain xylene, a neurotoxin. As with other products, that chemical odor is a clue that the product is giving off toxic fumes.

You may be aware that CFL light bulbs save you on your energy bill but contain mercury. This means you have to be very careful about disposing of them and you don't want to put them anywhere that there is a risk of them breaking. If you have a lamp that your kids might bump, use a different kind of bulb. Fortunately LED bulbs are now available and are even better for your energy bill without the risk of mercury. If you should break one of these CFL bulbs on a hard surface, do NOT try to sweep it up with your broom or vacuum. Open the windows to allow the mercury vapor to disperse, turn off fans and heaters, put on disposable gloves, clean up the droplets with an eyedropper and put them in a zip-lock bag. When you are done, put the eyedropper and the gloves in the bag. Put the bag inside another zip-lock bag and contact your local health department about how to dispose of it plus anything else (such as your clothing) the mercury may have come in contact with. If it is hard to clean up (such as in your carpet), contact a hazardous materials contractor to clean it up.

Eliminating as much as dust as possible from your home helps remove dust mites that can trigger allergies as well as the toxins found in house dust. Dust frequently using a non-toxic dusting spray. Vacuum carpets using a vacuum with a HEPA filter. Damp mop hard floors. Change your air filters every three months and use good HEPA ones that filter out dust, bacteria and mold spores.

One other toxin that may be found in your home is mold. Starting in the 1970's paint manufacturers began adding fungicide to paint in order to prevent mold. Unfortunately, this had the effect of creating mutations in molds. Our immune systems mount a greater immune response to the mutated forms so that we have more of a reaction. There is also a genetic component to our reaction to mold. People who carry certain versions of the HLA gene (histocompatibility locus A) are the ones who are likely to get sick. This is most common in people of

English, Irish, French, Welsh, German or Spanish ancestry. So while anyone can react to mold, about 25% of the population carries the genetic predisposition and will be more sensitive.

According to Dr. Richie Shoemaker, a physician who has become an expert in mold, symptoms that are associated with mold toxicity include

- Fatigue
- Weakness
- Aches
- Muscle Cramps
- Unusual Pain
- Ice Pick Pain
- Headache
- Light Sensitivity
- Red Eyes
- Blurred Vision
- Tearing
- Sinus Problems
- Cough
- Shortness of Breath
- Abdominal Pain
- Diarrhea
- Joint Pain
- Morning Stiffness
- Memory Issues
- Focus/Concentration Issues
- Word Recollection Issues
- Decreased Learning of New Knowledge
- Confusion
- Disorientation

- Skin Sensitivity
- Mood Swings
- Appetite Swings
- Sweats (especially night sweats)
- Temperature Regulation or Dysregulation Problems
- Excessive Thirst
- Increased Urination
- Static Shocks
- Numbness
- Tingling
- Vertigo
- Metallic Taste
- Tremors

Sometimes other illnesses are diagnosed when the underlying problem causing the symptoms is actually mold illness. Some of these diagnoses are:

- Fibromyalgia
- Chronic Fatigue Syndrome
- Multiple Sclerosis
- Depression
- Stress
- Allergy
- Post-Traumatic Stress Disorder
- Somatization
- Irritable Bowel Syndrome
- Attention Deficit Disorder

If you have one of these diagnoses and suspect your problem may be due to mold, your healthcare provider can do tests to check this out. If your healthcare provider is not familiar with mold problems and is unwilling to do the research, you may have to look for a specialist.

If you have mold problems, you need to find any ways that water is getting into your house and fix those. Then you need to get rid of porous surfaces that are affected such as carpeting. You don't have to get rid of your clothing because that can be washed. Children's' squeezable bath toys probably have mold inside them. Basements and attics are common places to find mold. Non porous surfaces can be cleaned with soap and water and then sprayed with straight vinegar. If you have extensive mold, you will need to hire experts to get rid of it but you can handle small amounts on your own. Generally fixing your current home is better than simply trying to move because chances are, the new home will also have issues. Dehumidifiers are also helpful in keeping your home less susceptible to mold growth.

House plants can be useful to improve the air quality of your home. They can actually filter out some of those VOCs. A potted plant for every 100 square feet is recommended (although you can't have too many). Some top rated plants for this include:

- English Ivy removes benzene, carbon monoxide, formaldehyde, trichloroethylene and mold.
- Peace Lily removes formaldehyde, benzene and trichloroethylene.
- Bamboo Palm removes formaldehyde.
- Ficus can remove pollutants from carpets.
- Dracaena helps remove the chemicals found in lacquers, varnishes and gasoline.

- Chrysanthemums help filter the chemicals found in glues, paints, detergents and plastics.
- Golden Pothos helps remove formaldehyde.
- Snake Plant is also known as mother-in-law's tongue and is a good choice for bathrooms since it tolerates low light and filters out the chemicals found in toilet paper and tissues.
- Spider Plants filter out chemicals from leather and rubber.
- Aloe Vera removes chemicals from paints and cleaning products.

Keep house plants out of the reach of pets and small children since some of them can be toxic if eaten. Some animals seem to know this as my beagle is only going after my basil and my goats would devour roses but never touch daffodils. Like everything, read up on your house plants.

In summary:
- Avoid flame retardants and anti-stain chemicals.
- Go for natural and organic materials in upholstered furniture and mattresses as much as possible.
- If you cannot replace your mattress that contains toxins, wrap it in polyethylene and use an organic cotton pad.
- Use real wood instead of manufactured wood products whenever possible.
- Use less toxic stains, paints and varnishes.
- Choose less toxic flooring options.
- Avoid PVC when possible.
- Replace lightbulbs with LEDs.
- Look for and treat mold if it is present.

- Dust and vacuum frequently and change air filters every three months. Use HEPA filters.
- Have lots of house plants to help filter the air.

Chapter Five

What to Wear

When you are thinking of toxins in your environment, clothing and fabrics are probably not the first thing that comes to mind. Once upon a time, clothing was made of cotton, wool, silk and linen. Now, clothing is either completely synthetic or synthetics are blended with the natural fibers. After all, who doesn't want permanent press, stain resistant clothing? Personally, I hate ironing so was delighted with permanent press clothing for many years and have to confess, I still have these fabrics in my closet. I completely understand why many people prefer to live in blissful ignorance about the many toxins we are exposed to everyday because once you know about these things, you can't unlearn them and you feel compelled to start making different choices.

Synthetic fabrics include acrylic, acetate, nylon, polyester, rayon and triacetate. Nylon and polyester are made from petrochemicals and their production creates nitrous oxide, a greenhouse gas that is 310 times more potent than carbon dioxide. Polyester is also known as Terylene, Dacron, Lycra or Vycron. Polyester emits phytoestrogens so is an endocrine disruptor and can promote the growth of cancer. It is associated with skin rashes, respiratory disorders and reduced sperm counts. It is also an environmental pollutant. Lycra or Spandex also contains polyurethane produced by mixing polyester with diisocyanate. It is then treated with stabiizers and other chemicals that can often trigger allergic reactions. Nylon retains chemical residues including formaldehyde, VOCs and fabric softening agents that can cause dermatitis, hyperpigmentation and central nervous system effects.

Acrylics are polycrylonitriles which may be carcinogenic. The EPA indicates that the effects of these chemicals is similar to cyanide, if inhaled, so workers who manufacture it can experience anemia, nausea, jaundice and kidney effects. It can irritate the skin and has been linked to breast cancer. Acetate and triacetate are made of cellulose from wood fibers which have had extensive chemical processing. You don't want to do your nails while wearing acetate as fingernail polish remover or polish will make it dissolve.

Rayon is made from wood pulp treated with chemicals like carbon disulphide, chlorine, caustic soda and sulphuric acid. Carbon disulphide is emitted from rayon fabrics and can cause nausea, vomiting, headache, chest and muscle pain and insomnia. Tencel is a newer version of rayon that is made with a nontoxic solvent.

Chemicals are also used for other reasons such as a formaldehyde product that is applied with heat so that it becomes part of the fabric to prevent shrinking. Then there are petrochemical dyes plus dye fixatives that are of special concern because they contain a host of toxic chemicals including heavy metals and bond with the fibers so that the clothing is color fast. This means they don't wash out. Both of these pollute water systems. Various chemicals are used to make clothing softer, wrinkle-free, moth repellant and stain-resistant. These chemicals have been linked to cancer, immune system damage, behavioral problems and hormone disruption. You have no doubt heard that Teflon is carcinogenic. This is because it contains perfluorinated chemicals (PFCs). It turns out that PFCs are also being added to clothing to make it last longer and to make it wrinkle-free. There are about 80,000 chemicals used by the textile industry and most of these have never been tested for human or environmental safety. Another problem is that even if a chemical is banned in your country, it may not be banned in the country where the clothing is produced. With so many textile jobs being outsourced to Asia where environmental regulations are more lax, you don't know what you are getting. For example, nonylphenol ethoxylates (NPEs) are banned in Europe but these are commonly used as detergents in the textile industry so are found in clothing that is imported from other countries.

Since the chemicals found in clothing are not going to be found on labels, there is not a lot of point in trying to list them all. Just be aware that synthetics, synthetic blends or anything that has been treated to make it wrinkle-resistant, stain resistant, static resistant or moth repellant will contain toxins. Nearly all fabrics, even organic ones, are treated with chemicals at some point but the natural fibers are much better choices so look for:

- Cotton, preferably organic
- Bamboo
- Hemp
- Linen
- Silk
- Wool

Cotton seeds are usually treated with fungicides or insecticides. Herbicides are applied to kill weeds as the plants are growing and cotton is heavily treated with insecticides. The nine most common pesticides are highly toxic and five are probably carcinogens. These can include Aldrin, Dieldren and DDT. Because cotton uses so many pesticides, it contaminates groundwater and soil. Let me also mention that you do not want to eat foods containing cottonseed oil.

Even organic cotton is treated with chemicals during the manufacturing process including detergents, brighteners, bleaches, softeners and dyes but is certainly an improvement over conventional. One thing I was not aware of was that cotton actually comes in different colors so organic "color-grown" cotton is a great alternative if you can find it.

Bamboo is a newcomer to the textile industry but can be grown sustainably without pesticides. It is similar to silk and cashmere in softness.

Hemp deserves special mention as it is not as familiar to most people. The hemp plant is related to the marijuana plant but does not contain significant amounts of THC, the substance found in marijuana that causes a "high". So, it has no use as a drug. It grows quickly and so close together that it chokes out weeds so doesn't require herbicides. It has been used in the past to make paper and rope but then was banned in the U.S. because of its relationship to marijuana and because it was a competitor to the emerging timber industry. In fact, it is far more sustainable than timber and has lots of uses. The one that we are looking at here is fabric because it can be used to make a variety of types of fabrics. It can also be used to replace plastic and to make hempcrete, a building material that is similar to concrete but non-toxic. Most of the hemp used in the U.S. is imported from Europe, Asia and Canada but laws are changing to allow cultivation of this useful plant in the U.S.

Linen comes from the inner bark of the flax plant and was widely used in the past. It is easier to grow organically than cotton and can be processed with less chemicals. If you have ever worn linen clothing, I'm sure you noticed that it wrinkles easily but is durable.

Silk is produced by silkworms when they spin their cocoons. In the past, it was grown without chemicals but then it was discovered that it was possible to extend the life of the silkworm with chemicals so that a bigger cocoon was produced and that killing the silkworm before it emerged from the cocoon led to more fibers. So, it may contain chemical additives unless it is wild-crafted.

Soy is another new product made from the soybeans. It is produced from the residue from making tofu, is soft and has been on the market since 2003.

Wool is generally produced from the fleece of sheep but there are other types as well.
- Alpaca fleece
- Mohair from the Angora goat
- Angora wool from the Angora rabbit
- Camel hair from the undercoat of the camel

- Cashmere from the down of the Kasmir goat
- Vicuna which is related to the llama

Conventional wool comes from sheep who may have been given hormones and antibiotics and dipped in organophosphate pesticides. The wool is then treated with detergents and toxic solvents. It is possible to get organic wool, which is preferable. Most of this comes from Australia. The amount produced will increase with consumer demand.

Often silk and wool clothing is labeled "dry clean only". Since conventional dry cleaning uses highly toxic chemicals such as perchloroethylene, a carcinogen and other chemicals that may be neurotoxic and damaging to the liver and kidneys as well as carcinogenic, it is best to avoid these dry cleaners. If you do dry clean something, remove the plastic bag and hang it outside so that the toxins can off gas. There are some environmental dry cleaners that do not use these highly toxic substances.

Often clothing with a dry cleaning label CAN be washed. You just have to use cold water and either hand wash or use the delicate cycle on the washer, then air dry. If I don't feel I can hand wash something with a dry clean only label, I don't buy it.

Bedding and towels should also be made of natural fibers. Organic cotton and wool are the best choices. Wash them before using to remove any fabric finishes.

One other consideration when buying clothing or other fabrics for your home. Look at the labels regarding where you clothing was made. You will notice that most clothing is now produced in Asia, Mexico or Central America. These countries have much less stringent environmental laws and less worker protections. So the people making your clothing are working under terrible conditions where they are probably exposed to toxic chemicals, working long hours and for a very small wage. Some of them may be children. This is because multinational corporations are trying to produce clothing as cheaply as possible so that they can make a bigger profit. If you have ethical concerns about this, look for clothing that is produced locally and/or buy used clothing so you are not contributing to the demand for cheap, foreign made clothing. By supporting thrift stores, you can also support good causes in your community.

In summary:
- Buy clothing and other fabric items made of natural fibers rather than synthetic ones.
- Buy organic when possible.
- Hand wash delicate fibers in cold water rather than dry cleaning them.
- Buy used.
- Buy local.

Chapter Six

Plastic: It is Everywhere

It is impossible to avoid plastic. It is versatile and cheap so is used to make all kinds of things that were once made of natural products such as glass, wood and metal. There are about 45 different types of plastics and these types contain variations. Here are some of the main ones you will see.

PETE

Polyethylene Terephthalate (PET or PETE) is labeled with the recycling number 1. It is often used for food storage and water bottles. It has been approved as safe by the FDA and can be recycled. It should not be reused. Recent studies have shown that PET can break down over time and leach into beverages in the bottle. The toxin DEHA has been found in water samples from reused water bottles and this toxin can cause liver and reproductive problems. It can also leach phthalates. It should not be subjected to heat or sunlight.

HDPE

High-density polyethylene (HDPE) is also used to make bottles and is used for milk bottles along with containers for other household products. It is also used to make items such as pipes, buckets and crates. It is identified by the recycling number 2 and is considered one of the safer plastics.

V

Polyvinyl chloride (PVC or vinyl) as previously discussed, can be used for building materials such as pipe, siding window frames fencing and decking. It can also be produced in a flexible form to make shower curtains, shrink wrap and deli wrap. The FDA states that vinyl chloride, a component of PVC, is a human carcinogen but that the amount used in food packaging is within safe limits. There is a plasticizer called DEHP found in some PVC including the type used for medical bags. DEHP has been linked to cancer and other ill effects in lab animals so that people undergoing invasive medical procedures may have been exposed to levels higher than what is safe; the FDA has recommended that this be removed or at least labeled. PVC is labeled as recycling number 3 on household products.

Production of PVC requires toxic chemicals like chlorine and vinyl chloride plus toxic additives to make the PVC stable. These additives include phthalates, lead, cadmium and tin. The EPA proposed standards in 2000 to limit the toxic emissions from PVC production plants.

LDPE

Low-density polyethylene (LDPE) is number 4 and is used to make bottles that require extra flexibility such as squeezable bottles. It is also used for the coating on milk cartons, grocery bags, garbage bags, shrink wrap, toys, container lids and packaging.

Polypropylene (PP) has a high melting point so it is useful for hot liquids that are cooled in a bottle like syrup or ketchup. It can be flexible or rigid and is used for margarine, yogurt and take-out containers. It can also be used for medicine bottles, bottle caps and other items. It uses less toxic additives during manufacture. It is labeled number 5.

Polystyrene (PS) or styrene is most often used for Styrofoam. You have seen it in protective packaging for delicate items and food service packaging like cups and meat trays. It is also used for foam insulation. It is number 6 although it is not considered recyclable. Styrene is a carcinogen and also out gases phthalates. It should not be used as a food container.

Recycling number 7 is for all other types of plastics including **polycarbonates.** These are hard and durable and often used for reusable water bottles. These can leach BPA so are not a good choice. We discussed them in the chapter on water.

Another highly toxic plastic is **polytetrafluoroethylene**, otherwise known as **Teflon**. It can cause cancer and birth defects in animals and may pose the same threat to humans. When heated to high temperatures, it can release toxic fumes. Birds are very sensitive to this and it has resulted in the death of many pet birds. It can cause flu-like symptoms in humans. If you are still using Teflon pans, I suggest you replace them.

There is no such thing as a good plastic but the ones you will especially want to avoid are numbers 3, 6 and 7 as these are the most toxic. Try to buy things in glass or paper containers rather than plastic. Especially when it comes to food, avoid plastics and cans when you can and **never heat food in any kind of plastic container**. Buy glass containers to put your leftovers in. Invest in some good pots and pans that don't have Teflon. I have stainless steel waterless cookware that is guaranteed to last and is easy to clean. Use cloth grocery bags; I have some that fold up in my purse so I am never without them. Any time you have a choice between plastic and a natural product such as wood, glass, ceramic or metal, go for the natural stuff. It is now possible to buy disposable items such as cups made of compostable natural products such as corn. Just about anything made from plastic can also be made from hemp. If consumers demand these products, we can reduce the amount of plastic produced.

When you do use plastic, recycle it so it doesn't end up in a landfill while increasing the need to manufacture more plastic. Remember that it is a petrochemical so it is made from oil. Extraction and use of fossil fuels is driving global warming plus plastic does not biodegrade and will be with us for centuries. It is killing fish in the ocean who eat it and get tangled in it. The people who manufacture it are exposed to even more toxins than the consumers who use it. Your recycling company can let you know what types of plastics it is willing to take. You can count on them taking PET and HDPE but some companies will take others as well.

In summary:

- Try not to buy things made of plastic or packaged in plastic.
- Purchase food in glass containers rather than plastic or cans whenever possible.
- Buy glass containers for storing food.
- Never heat food in plastic.
- Don't use cookware with Teflon.
- Use reusable, cloth grocery bags.
- If you are using disposable products, try to find ones that can be composted rather than plastic ones.
- Recycle plastic that you do use as much as possible.

Chapter Seven
Energy

We use energy to heat and cool our homes, to run all kinds of appliances and electrical devices, for cooking, for heating water, for powering our vehicles and assorted tools like lawnmowers and saws. And then we are exposed to electromagnetic field (EMF) radiation as a result of all the electrical and technological devices that we are surrounded with but before we deal with that, let's look at how you are powering everything.

Let's start with heating. If you burn oil, gas, kerosene, propane, coal or wood for heating and/or cooking, you are causing indoor air pollution. Burning these fuels can give off carbon monoxide and nitrogen dioxide. Nitrogen dioxide is a reddish brown gas that is irritating to the eyes and throat. Carbon monoxide is an odorless, colorless gas that can displace the oxygen in your blood stream. It can cause headaches, dizziness, fatigue, confusion and disorientation. If you are using a combustion source heater, you should have a carbon monoxide detector (similar to a smoke alarm). Any sort of combustion heater should be inspected periodically to make sure it is working properly. If you see a yellow-tipped flame in a stove or gas space heater, that is a sign that not all of the fuel is being burned completely and that you are giving off pollutants. If you are burning wood, you may also be giving off ash, which is hard on your lungs. Do not burn pressure treated wood since it has been treated with chemicals that will be released when it is burned. Have fireplace chimneys cleaned and inspected. Unvented space heaters running

73

off gas or kerosene are especially dangerous to use indoors and require that you open a window or door to allow the gases to escape.

If you are using electric heat, you are avoiding polluting gases in your home but the energy company that you purchase electricity from may be doing the polluting for you. In the area where I live, a coal plant has been causing air pollution (the levels of nitrogen dioxide have been a particular concern) and pollution of water from leaking coal ash ponds. It is to be replaced by a natural gas plant but the production of natural gas is generally done by fracking, which causes the release of methane gas and often contaminates that ground water in the area. Methane is an even greater contributor to global warming than the carbon dioxide that results from the burning of fossil fuels. Check with your energy company to see if they offer a green option where by paying a few dollars more, they will get the amount of energy that you are using from green power such as solar or wind. There are also energy companies such as Arcadia that generate power via wind. You can purchase your energy from them and they coordinate this with your local power company.

Another option is to purchase or lease solar panels and generate your own electricity. In some cases, during times that you are producing more electricity than you are using, your electricity goes back to the power company and they pay you or credit you for that electrical power. You can also receive tax credits for switching to green energy. If you are not connected to an energy company, you are "off-grid" and will need a battery system to store energy produced so that it is available when the system is not generating electricity. For example, when the sun is shining, your solar panels will not only provide energy for using immediately but will store excess energy so that it is available at night when none is being produced.

Other sources of heating and cooling include geothermal. A ground source heat pump relies on the fact that the temperature below ground remains fairly constant all year. By running pipes with liquid below the ground, heat from a building is cooled during the summer and heat from the ground is used to warm the building during the winter. Especially in areas with temperature extremes, geothermal can be one of the most efficient ways to heat and cool a house. The heat pump generates 3 to 5 times more energy than is required to run it. Drawbacks are the upfront costs to dig up the area around the house to install it but it generally pays for itself in 8 to 12 years. It is becoming increasingly popular and is a good alternative in rural areas where natural gas is not available and electricity may be expensive. Geothermal can also be used for power plants and we may be seeing more of this in the future as we move away from fossil fuels to renewable energy.

You might want to check with your power company to see if they do energy audits. Some companies do these for free and this allows you to see if there are changes you can make to reduce the amount of electricity you use. Some of these changes might be to improve insulation, put weather stripping around doors, using appliances that are more efficient, changing light bulbs to more efficient types such as LEDs, wrapping your water heater in an insulating blanket (or switching to a tankless water heater) and unplugging electrical appliances that are not in use.

Unplugging anything you are not currently using has an additional benefit of reducing electromagnetic field (EMF) radiation. Anything with electrical current as well as devices such as cell phones, WiFi, wireless modems, power lines and cell phone towers generate EMF radiation. Most people do not experience any symptoms from this but there has been increasing concern as our exposure has increased dramatically over the past couple of decades.

EMF radiation is non-ionizing radiation. Ionizing radiation is the kind found in x-rays, radon and other radioactive materials and that has been linked to cancer. We don't really know for sure what the health effects of EMFs are yet but it is wise to err on the side of caution. Our bodies have an electrical system that we use to send signals for biological functions so it is certainly possible for these EMFs to affect us. It has been proposed that long-term effects could include cancer, birth defects, chronic fatigue, immune system problems, cognitive and neurological disorders. More research is needed but so far, the possible dangers, raised in the research that has been done, have been downplayed.

Try to keep electrical items away from your bed since you spend a lot of time there. Put your electric clock across the room. If you use an electric blanket, use it to warm the bed before you get in, then unplug it.

There has been some research on the dangers of cell phones showing that there is a possible increase in cancer along with other ill effects but this has been largely ignored. If you have a cell phone (and almost all of us do), try to limit use and keep it farther away from your body. The EMF drops to one fourth the strength at a distance of two inches and is fifty times lower at three feet. Get one with the lowest possible SAR (Specific Absorption Rate) which is a measure of the strength of the magnetic field absorbed by the body. Young children and pregnant women should be especially cautious.

We haven't talked about cars yet but gasoline powered cars are a huge contributor to air pollution, giving off the same gases as other types of combustion. Fortunately, we now have quite a few choices of hybrid and electric vehicles which are improving all the time. People with respiratory illnesses such as asthma and COPD will benefit greatly from the switch away from vehicles powered by fossil fuels.

An even worse polluter than your car is your gasoline powered lawn mower. Using a gasoline lawn mower for an hour is the pollution equivalent of driving 40 cars for an hour. Large lawns and those big ride-on mowers are terrible for the environment. If you do have grass, you might want to investigate using a scythe or old fashioned push mower. I recently got an Austrian scythe and find that easier to use on wet or taller grass than a mower.

All the chemicals used to keep those lawns green and weed free leach into the water so affect all of us. If you have a large piece of land, you can create a much more interesting landscape with the use of trees, shrubs and other plants that require less care than lawn. I would also suggest that you consider growing your own food. You can intersperse flowers with your vegetables which attracts pollinators and, in some cases, protects against harmful insects while making your garden more colorful and pleasing to the eye. Learn how to use mulch and compost to produce healthy soil and plants without the use of chemicals. Mulch can reduce your need to water as often and help control unwanted plants (weeds). Composting is a way to take your yard waste (such as dead leaves) and kitchen scraps to produce healthy soil and plants. Gardening is good exercise and is good for mental health besides providing the benefit of organic food.

In summary:

- Try to use efficient, non-polluting sources of energy to heat and cool your home.
- Be sure to get any combustion type heating source checked periodically and install a carbon monoxide monitor.
- Try to reduce your use of energy.
- Use energy efficient lighting and appliances.
- Use insulation to improve energy efficiency of your home.
- Check with your power company about an energy audit.
- Disconnect and unplug electrical devices when not in use.
- Limit cell phone use and keep it farther away from your body.
- Consider a hybrid or electric vehicle.

- Reduce or eliminate your lawn.
- Consider replacing it with food producing plants such as fruit trees, berry bushes and vegetable gardens.
- Learn to use mulch and compost.
- Avoid using chemicals in your yard. If you need to kill a weed, use straight vinegar to spray it instead of Round-Up. It may take several applications but it is safe. Boiling water or devices that burn the weed also work.

Chapter Eight
Medical Care

Standard medical care does some things very well. Trauma care and surgical procedures are things that we do well. The treatment and prevention of chronic disease leave a lot to be desired.

In the United States, good healthcare is impaired by the stranglehold that the pharmaceutical companies have on our government. Heavy lobbying by these companies has resulted in exorbitant prices for drugs and for their infiltration into management of the very agencies, such as the FDA (Federal Drug Administration) that are supposed to regulate them. As a result, new medications are approved based on the testing done by the pharmaceutical company that created them, the companies are protected by patents so generic versions cannot be created for many years and the prices of the drug in this country are higher than the same drug in other countries. In some cases, drugs have come on to the market and are later found to be unsafe but meanwhile the company which produced them has made a lot of money. Some well-known examples include Vioxx, an arthritis drug that doubled the risk of heart attacks and strokes, Phen-fen, a diet drug that caused heart damage, and Propulsid, a drug to reduce stomach acid that also caused heart damage.

The FDA reports adverse reactions to drugs that they have approved annually. A serious reaction is one that results in death, hospitalization, disability, congenital anomaly, is life-threating or other serious reaction. These have been increasing over time and have gone from 153,818 serious reactions of which 19,445 resulted in death in the year 2000 to 471,291 serious reactions and 82,724 deaths in 2010. If you watch American television, I'm sure you have seen advertisements for medications. Pay attention to the list of side effects. Before taking any prescription medication, discuss the benefits and risks with your healthcare provider including whether there might be an older, safer drug you could use. Be informed about side effects and only take medications when needed.

Medications for pain are a particular problem due to deaths from overdoses. Of the 38,329 drug overdose deaths in the U.S. in 2010, 22,134 were the result of pharmaceutical drugs with the most common (75%) being opioids (narcotics such as hydrocodone and oxycodone). Others include benzodiazepines (like Valium and Xanax), antidepressants, antiepileptic and antiparkinsonian drugs, especially when used in combination. Over-the-counter pain medications also have risks. Each year non-steroidal anti-inflammatory drugs (NSAIDs), such as aspirin, Motrin and Naproxen, cause about 7,600 deaths and 76,000 hospitalizations in the United States. Acetaminophen (Tylenol) can cause liver damage/toxicity leading to 458 deaths between 1996 and 1998.

Pharmaceutical companies spend a lot on prescribers and future prescribers by contributing to medical schools and by providing continuing education and having drug representatives call on doctors to give them samples of new drugs and encourage prescribing of their drug. In order to make money, doctors spend as little time as possible with patients so they can see more patients per day. It is much faster and easier to prescribe medication than to spend time teaching patients what they can do to improve their health. All drugs have side effects and sometimes people end up on multiple medications, some of which are to treat the side effects of other ones. Sometimes patients are started on samples of new drugs but then cannot afford to continue them because the price is so high or because the drug isn't covered by their insurance. I remember seeing a patient who was a single mom working in a fast food restaurant and having her tell me that she wasn't taking the drug her cardiologist prescribed (and told her she had to take) because she had to make a choice between the drug and feeding her children. Furthermore, she couldn't go back to see him about finding a cheaper drug because he dropped her when she couldn't pay her bill.

Insurance companies also play a role, in that payment is based on disease codes so the sicker the doctor can make you look on your medical record with multiple diagnoses, making you a complex patient, the better their reimbursement. So, if a doctor wants to make a good living, they see patients very quickly and diagnose and code for lots of problems for which you receive prescription medication. I worked in this system so know how this works. This does not give healthcare providers time to really listen to their patients and do the teaching necessary to help them make lifestyle changes. Physicians are given very little training on nutrition or other healthy lifestyle changes so this means they are not really prepared to help patients in this way. This means it is up to us to learn about our health on our own.

We need to recognize that pharmaceutical companies and insurance companies are based on making profits, not ensuring our good health. Those of you who live in countries with a national healthcare system don't have a lot of the problems that U.S. citizens do which is why you have better health with a lower per capita cost for healthcare. You have a system that is affordable and covers everyone. I hope that the U.S. will have that someday and that we will outlaw the outrageous lobbying that encourages our politicians to support policies that are not in the public interest.

Much of the illness and disability we suffer is due to chronic disease and much of this is due to lifestyle. As previously stated, your doctor hasn't had a lot of training in nutrition or exercise. He or she has learned how to order tests, make diagnoses and prescribe pharmaceuticals. Even taking a good in-depth history from you and physical exam skills are not relied on as much as they were in the past. The research studies that are used to support various treatments are often sponsored by the pharmaceutical company or by a university that is receiving funding from them and your busy healthcare provider keeps up with the current knowledge from reading a few medical journals or from the information from drug reps. This is the standard medical model used by allopathic (mainstream) physicians.

There is now a newer branch of medicine called functional or holistic medicine that looks at underlying causes of illness and uses a broader approach to treatment. In some cases, this means looking at older plant based treatments. It definitely looks at nutrition as being an important part of health. Some mainstream healthcare providers are incorporating some of this into their practices. One of the problems is that research studies may not be available on some of the herbal and nutraceutical therapies because these studies are expensive and supplement manufacturers are unable to afford them. Universities are doing more research in this area because of patients using these products. For example, Vitamin D has been heavily studied in recent years so that there is plenty of research showing us that many people are deficient in this Vitamin and that lower levels are linked to many diseases.

On the other hand, there are a lot of people trying to cash in on the interest in supplements that push their version of various supplements. When you hear someone who is selling vitamins and supplements tell you how their product is a miracle cure and giving you case studies of how it helped Bill and Jennifer, take these with a grain of salt. Like medications, do your research so that you are not wasting your money.

Vaccines are an issue of great controversy. Vaccinations are heavily pushed by the U.S. government and by the companies that manufacture them. We are told that they are safe and effective. There is no question that the number of cases of vaccine-preventable diseases has plummeted since vaccinations have been introduced but they are not without some risks.

Back in the 1970s and 1980s, there were a number of lawsuits against vaccine manufacturers, mostly about the DPT vaccine and oral polio vaccine. So, the pharmaceutical companies asked for, and got, protection against liability. This means that you cannot sue them for any injury resulting from a vaccine. The 1986 National Child Injury Act sets up a special court system that is able to award compensation. These claims generally take years to go through the court system and two-thirds of them are denied. There is also a Vaccine Adverse Event Reporting System (VAERS) which reports that there are about 5,000 deaths per year. The International Medical Council on Vaccination (IMCV) estimates that 3,900 of the deaths are directly attributable to vaccines. Since not all adverse reactions or deaths may be reported to VAERS, the number is probably quite a bit higher. Dr. David Kessler, a former head of the FDA, stated that he thought the reporting rate might only be around 1% which would mean that there could be as many as 39,000 vaccine-related deaths per year. So, while most people have no problems with vaccination, we need to be aware that they are not as safe as we are being told.

Besides deaths, there are a number of other possible adverse effects. Common side effects are pain at the injection site and mild fever. Anaphylaxis, a life-threatening allergic reaction is possible although rare. Other serious adverse effects include Guillian-Barre Syndrome, seizures and neurological disorders. The pertussis component of the DPT vaccine has especially been linked to encephalopathy so that DTaP vaccine which has an acellular pertussis was developed. The OPV (oral polio) vaccine has an attenuated or weakened form of live polio virus resulting in some cases of paralytic polio plus the shedding of live virus that could cause polio in immunocompromised contacts. This led to the use of IPV (inactivated polio virus).

The way vaccines work is to give you either a killed or weakened strain of a virus so that your body will develop an immune response to it. This is only one part of your body's immune response to foreign invaders and the response to a vaccine only provides a temporary form of immunity. This is why booster shots are given. Exposure to the disease itself generally produces life-long immunity.

In addition to the killed or weakened (attenuated) form of the virus, vaccines contain adjuvants. One of these is aluminum, which is added to enhance the immune response. While we do get aluminum in our food and water, these are small amounts and very little is absorbed. When aluminum is injected, your body gets all of it. Infant kidneys are not good at removing aluminum and since babies are getting a lot more aluminum containing vaccines than they received in the past (up to 4,925 mcg in the first 18 months), this is of concern. Aluminum is a neurotoxin which is ingested by macrophages (immune cells) in your body and these are able to carry it across the blood brain barrier.

Vaccines can also contain preservatives. Thimerosal was used in quite a few vaccines in the past but in 1999, the US Public Health Service recommended removing it because it contains mercury. It is now found only in vaccines from multi-dose vials such as the flu vaccines.

Other substances may be found in vaccines. These include antibiotics used in manufacturing of the vaccine, formaldehyde and phenol which are used to inactivate viruses and detoxify bacterial toxins, sugars, amino acids and proteins that may be added as stabilizers and fetal calf serum used to grow the virus for manufacture into a vaccine. The safety of some of these (especially formaldehyde and phenol) is questionable.

The effectiveness of vaccines can be questionable. In a virus which mutates rapidly such as influenza, a flu shot against particular strains does not protect you against other strains. Each year scientists try to guess which strains are likely to be active in the upcoming flu season (late fall and winter). One way to do this is to look at what strains are active in the winter in the Southern hemisphere to try to determine what strains will be active in the Northern hemisphere when winter arrives there. Then these strains are used to manufacture a vaccine. Sometimes they guess correctly and other years they are wrong and the flu vaccine turns out to be useless or only partially effective.

Pertussis is another virus which has mutated so that while the vaccine may reduce the symptoms in people who have been vaccinated, they can still be infected and transmit the disease to others. It is possible to have no symptoms and spread the disease. There are undoubtedly many cases that are never diagnosed. When someone has a persistent cough without a known cause, pertussis should be considered. The mumps vaccine may be another one that is not that effective. There has been a recent outbreak of mumps on a college campus and all of those diagnosed had been vaccinated against mumps.

If you are contemplating getting pregnant and want to be vaccinated, it is better to do it prior to becoming pregnant. Many vaccines which were not given to pregnant women in the past, are now being encouraged during pregnancy but since an unborn child is much more sensitive to toxins than an adult, you might want to be cautious about this.

One of the things you can do to protect yourself against the flu and other viral illnesses is to improve your own body's immune response. I don't get flu shots and despite plenty of exposures, have only had the flu twice in my life and both of those were many years ago. I consider having a level of Vitamin D of at least 50 (determined by blood test) to be more effective than a flu shot. Since this protects against other illnesses besides the flu and helps against all flu strains, not just the ones in the current flu shot, this seems to me to be a better choice.

Having a better immune system even helps protect you against cancer. Cancer is a mutation of normal cells into cancerous ones. This is a normal occurrence but generally a healthy body is able to eliminate abnormal cells. This means having a normal immune system. We know that although there are some genetic factors that can put some people at risk for certain cancers, a huge factor in the development of cancer is your exposure to environmental toxins and your general health also plays a role. If you are, like so many people these days, overweight, diabetic and prone to catching every illness that comes around, your risk of getting cancer is higher. I hope the information in this book will help you reduce your exposure to toxins and also encourage good health habits that will change this.

Once someone is diagnosed with cancer, they are generally given three options, usually a combination of them. These are surgery, chemotherapy and radiation. Usually there is no mention of nutrition or alternative therapies. What you need to know is that surgery is stressful, chemotherapy is a toxin that is extremely hard on your immune system and radiation is known to cause cancer even though a large dose to a tumor will kill those cells. This is not to say that these approaches are not useful but if you want to get rid of cancer and not have it return, you need to address more than just the identified cancer cells. You have to improve your health so that your body can fight the cancer. Treatment for cancer that diminishes your immune response can result in the return of cancer.

Cancer cells are more metabolically active than normal cells. Chemotherapy works because the cancer cells will take up the toxic drug faster than the normal cells so that they will be more likely to be killed than the rest of your cells. Because it is a toxin, your health suffers and you have horrible side effects. If you feel like you are being poisoned, it is because you are. Doctors monitor white blood cells (part of your immune system) and if they fall too low, they have to hold off on the next dose of chemo. This is why many people, when told that the disease is going to be fatal, will choose to forgo a few extra months of life being ill with chemo, knowing that the quality of the time left is more important than the quantity.

Did you know that sugar promotes the growth of cancer? By using insulin to drop the blood sugar, the dose of the chemotherapy drug can be reduced so that there are less side effects. You can use diet to drop your blood sugar and help to prevent cancer (and help treat it, if you are already diagnosed with it). Nutrition is critical if you want to have a body healthy enough to fight cancer. Lots of vegetables, especially leafy greens are especially helpful. A diet of fresh, whole and organic food and avoidance of the ones that raise blood sugar can be used to prevent, help treat and prevent recurrence of cancer.

There are many alternative treatments that can be used to fight cancer and it is worthwhile to do some research on these. One that is in the news right now is CBD oil. This comes from the hemp plant, a relative of marijuana, which is beginning to be grown in the U.S. again after being banned for many years. It is certainly worth looking at all of your options.

Diabetes and obesity are epidemic right now, largely as a result of our poor diet, lack of activity and exposure to toxins. My book, *Lose Weight without Hunger* discusses ways to use the glycemic index to reduce blood sugar and lose weight. If you have a sedentary job, get up every 30 minutes or so and move around. Find activities that you enjoy that increase the amount of activity you get. You don't have to join a gym unless you enjoy that. You can garden and grow some of your own food. You can get a dog and take it for walks. You can go out dancing. The main thing is to find something that gives you pleasure and gives you activity. This helps reduce your stress level and that reduces cortisol, a hormone that is especially good at producing abdominal fat. Both obesity and a sedentary lifestyle are linked to type 2 diabetes.

We haven't talked about mental health but lifestyle is important here too. Did you know that getting outdoors in the sunshine and walking (or engaging in some sort of activity) is as effective for depression as antidepressants? A good diet, activity, avoiding toxins, meditation and getting enough sleep will do wonders for your mental health. To address all of these would require another book and if depression is an issue for you, you might want to read *A Mind of Your Own* by Kelly Brogan, MD. Make sure that you have fun and opportunities for laughter as a regular part of your life.

Most of us do not get enough sleep and it seems to be considered a good thing in our culture if you can get by with only four to six hours of sleep. Actually, this is detrimental to your health. You need at least seven hours of sleep and most of us need eight. The blue spectrum light from TV and computer screens tends to keep you awake so turn them off before you want to fall asleep. Try reading a book or some other quiet activity so you can get to sleep earlier.

I generally recommend that everyone take a good quality probiotic, have their Vitamin D level tested and supplement accordingly (generally 2,000 to 5,000 IUs of Vitamin D3 is needed to keep the level above 50) and other vitamins, minerals and supplements as needed. The use of commercial fertilizers and glyphosate has left our soil in poor condition so that we do not always get the nutrition from our food that we need. The B vitamins and vitamin C are water soluble so that your body will excrete them in your urine if you take more than you need but these are necessary as co-enzymes for necessary chemical reactions. Most of us are deficient in magnesium so I often suggest that patients take magnesium citrate rather than the common magnesium sulfate for better adsorption. I also recommend fish oil and ubiquinol (the effective form of Co-Enzyme Q 10). Finding a naturopathic or holistic physician is the best way to come up with an individualized plan since that is not something I can address in a book. There are also other practitioners such as Chinese herbalists and acupuncturists who can help with some health problems.

I hope I have given you information that will help you make changes in your life leading to better health. We are constantly bombarded with messages from advertising to encourage us to eat and use things that can make our health worse. The best way to counter that is knowledge.

In summary:
- Recognize that you need to take responsibility for your own health rather than relying on government agencies to protect you or doctors to have the time to check out everything for you.
- Do your research and ask questions.

- Make lifestyle changes as needed.
- Seek out alternative health practitioners as needed.

Chapter Nine
In Conclusion

I thought I was fairly knowledgeable about environmental toxins before I started this book and was surprised to find how much I didn't know. I spent months reading tons of material from books, blog posts, web sites and articles from medical and scientific sources. I tried to read different points of view from doctors, scientists and passionate lay people who had taken the time to focus on and learn about a particular issue. I learned a tremendous amount and have tried to take all that I learned and condense it down into a concise, readable book that will enable anyone to recognize toxins in their environment and take steps to make changes that will limit their exposure to them.

Is it possible to avoid all toxins? Certainly not. We have always had some toxic substances in our environment and our body is able to deal with this. But now, in addition to natural substance that are toxic, we have large amounts man-made toxins. What we are trying to do is to reduce our exposure to them as much as is feasible so that we do not suffer ill health from them.

I had already made dietary changes so that most of the food I eat is organic. I also had long since discarded Teflon coated pans for stainless steel and switched from plastic food storage containers to glass ones. I had also switched to safer personal care products without things like parabens and phthalates. I has switched to a "green" laundry detergent, a safer dishwashing liquid and homemade cleaning products. I drive a hybrid car and try to plan my trips to save gasoline. I recycle and reuse things and drink filtered tap water. I tend to use supplements rather than prescription drugs. So I was already doing lots of the things I suggest in this book but found there were lots of other things I had not considered.

Since doing the research for this book, I replaced my mattress and am much more conscious of other things I buy. For example, I found a non-toxic wood sealer that I used on the wood to build my raised beds for my garden. I will be converting the lawn of the home I just purchased to gardens, bushes and trees that will provide food using permaculture principles and have no intention of buying a power mower. There are lots of small changes we can make as we replace things we use with safer alternatives and use new knowledge to make changes in our buying behavior.

I hope that, armed with knowledge from this book, you will find yourself making changes in what you buy. If you currently suffer from health problems that are aggravated by toxins in your environment, these should improve. If you have found this book useful, I hope you will leave a good review on Amazon and encourage your friends to read it. Should you want to learn more about any of the things covered in the book, check out the references. Wishing you good health.

References

Books:

Angell, Marcia, _The Truth About the Drug Companies: How They Deceive Us and What To Do About It_, Ballantine Books, 2005.

Black, Janet L., _Losing Weight Without Hunger_, Peaceful Heart Press, 2014.

Brogan, Kelly, M.D., A _Mind of Your Own_, Harper Wave, 2016.

Button, Kimberly, _The Everything Guide to a Healthy Home_, Adams Media, 2012.

Colborn, Theo; Dumanoski, Dianne; Myers, John Peterson; _Our Stolen Future_, Plume, 1997.

Davis, William, M.D. _Wheat Belly_, Rodale, Inc., 2011

Druker, Steven M., _Altered Genes, Twisted Truth_, Clear River Press, 2015.

Hari, Vani, _The Food Babe Way_, Little Brown and Company, 2015.

Lourie, Bruce and Smith, Rick, *Toxin Toxout,* St Martin's Press, 2013.

Mullin, Gerard E., *The Gut Balance Revolution,* Rodale, 2015.

Perlmutter, David, M.D., *Brain Maker,* Little, Brown and Company, 2015.
_____and Loberg, Kristan, *Grain Brain,* Little and Brown, 2013.

Shojai, Pedram, *The Urban Monk,* Rodale, 2016.

Smith, Jeffrey M. *Seeds of Deception,* Yes! Books, 2003.

Somers, Suzanne, *Tox-Sick,* Harmony Books, 2015.

Steingraber, Sandra, *Living Downstream,* Da Capo Press, 2010.

Steinman, David, *Safe Trip to Eden,* Thunder's Mouth Press, 2007.

Sharyn Wynters and Goldberg, Burton, *The Pure Cure,* Soft Skull Press, 2012.

Articles, blogs and web pages:

Chapter One:

Carman, Judy; Heinemann, Jack; and Agapito-Tenfen, Sarah; *New Paper on dsRNA Risks – briefing for non-specialists, 21 March 2013,* http://www.gmwatch.org.

_____, A comparative evaluation of the regulation of GM crops or products containing dsRNA and suggested improvements to risk assessments, *Environ. Int. 55,* 43-55, 2013.

Chapter Two:

www.activistpost.com/...13/04/7-tap-water-toxins.html

www.cdc.gov/drinking/public/drinking-water-faq.html

http://ecowatch.com/2015/07/16/bpa-in-canned-food.

Ferrer, Elaine Catherine and Cummins, Ronnie, *Hormone Disruptors: Everyday Poisons in Non-Organic Food, Body Care Products, water Bottles and Home Furniture,* Organic Consumers Association, April 13, 2016.

www.globalhealingcenter.com/water/water-toxins

www.healthguidance.org/...hat-Chemicals-Are-in-Tap.

https://www.epa.gov/dwstandardsregulations

www.ewg.org/...08/your-drinking-water-contaminated...

www.ewg.org/tap-water/reportfindings

articles.mercola.com/.../fluoride-drinking-water.aspx

www.scientificamerican.com/unregulated-chemicals-found-in...

Chapter Three:
chemistry.about.com/healthsafety/tp/toxic-chemicals-in...

daniwalker.com/toxins-in-personal-care-products

www.davidsuzuki.org/...dirty-dozen-cosmetic-chemicals

www.hsph.harvard.edu/...als-in-personal-care-products

www.healthychild.org/...n-your-personal-care-products

www.keeperofthehome.org/...ersonal-care-products.html

mamavation.com/removing-toxins-from-your-personal-care...

www.mercola.com/graphics/personal-care-products.htm

www.naturalnews.com/toxic
chemicals_personal_care_products.html

www.treehugger.com/20-toxic-care-products-and-cosmetics.html

www.webmd.com/.../personal-care-products

www.breastcancerfund.org/links/household-products

www.davidsuzuki.org/issues/health/science/toxics/the-dirt-on-toxic...

www.ewg.org/...s/cleaners/content/cleaners_and_health

www.foxnews.com/health/10-ways-to-rid-your-body-toxic...

www.thedailybeast.com/most-toxic-cleaning-products.html

www.webofcreation.org/...Toxins-cleaning products.htm

www.webmd.com/many-cleaning-products-said-to-contain-toxins

Chapter Four:

http://empoweredsustenance.com/toxic-mattress/

http://livewholebefree.com/wordpress/how-to-avoid-harmful-toxins-in-mattresses/

http://www.mattress-inquirer.com/do-you-have-a-toxic-mattress/

http://www.mommypotamus.com/how-to-buy-a-non-toxic-mattress/

http://www.motherjones.com/politics/2008/03/should-you-ditch-your-chemical-mattress

http://www.oprah.com/world/Tips-for-Buying-an-Eco-Friendly-Mattress

https://savvyrest.com/articles-research

http://www.sleepjunkie.org/are-memory-foam-mattresses-safe/

http://www.sustainablebabysteps.com/mattress-toxins.html

http://blackdoctor.org/14220/toxic-chemicals-in-furniture

http://eartheasy.com/live_reducing_indoor_toxins.html

www.getipm.com/articles/10-worst-hometoxins.htm

http://www.green-talk.com/are-toxic-chemicals-lurking-in-your-furniture-and-building-products/

http://www.healthextremist.com/toxic-furniture-in-your-home-affecting-health/

http://www.huffingtonpost.com/sarah-janssen/my-toxic-couch_b_2205073.html

http://life.gaiam.com/article/your-furniture-hazardous-your-health-4-lessons-learn-about-formaldehyde

http://www.medicaldaily.com/9-toxic-chemicals-found-furniture-your-home-hazard-zone-256572

www.organicauthority.com/toxins-in-your-home-room...

www.oprah.com/...ns-in-Your-Furniture-Making-You-Sick

http://pollutioninpeople.org/safer/products/furniture

http://www.sfgate.com/health/article/Chemicals-in-furniture-hard-to-avoid-4072857.php

http://www.theatlantic.com/health/archive/2014/09/how-to-test-a-couch-for-toxins/380823/

http://www.usatoday.com/story/news/nation/2012/11/28/couches-sofas-toxic-flame-retardants-chemicals/1729769/

http://www.cdc.gov/nceh/publications/books/housing/cha05.htm

http://eartheasy.com/live_reducing_indoor_toxins.html

http://www.emedicinehealth.com/environmental_illness-health/page3_em.htm

http://www.globalhealingcenter.com/health-hazards-to-know-about/industrial-chemical-toxins

http://healthybuildingscience.com/2012/11/27/toxic-building-materials-in-residential-construction/

http://www.huffingtonpost.com/2013/12/12/building-materials-asthma_n_4427243.html

http://www.nchh.org/Resources/Building-Materials-and-Products/Potential-Chemicals-Found-in-Building-Materials.aspx

http://www.sixwise.com/newsletters/06/08/16/the-five-home-construction-materials-that-pose-the-highest-health-risk-to-you.htm

http://www.isse.org.uk/toxins/toxins-in-paint/

http://www.journalnow.com/home_food/home_garden/d
iy/silent-dangers-traditional-paints-solvents-emit-harmful-
toxic-chemicals/article_4648cea8-8784-11e2-933c-
001a4bcf6878.html

http://www.motherearthnews.com/green-homes/toxic-
chemicals-in-paint-zmaz03onzgoe.aspx

http://www.cdc.gov/mold/stachy.htm

https://www.bulletproofexec.com/transcript-126-
surviving-mold-with-dr-ritchie-shoemaker/

https://www.epa.gov/mold

http://www.medicinenet.com/mold_exposure/article.htm

http://articles.mercola.com/sites/articles/archive/2011/09
/03/molds-making-you-ill.aspx

http://www.mold-help.org/

Chapter Five:
http://www.belmarrahealth.com/the-toxins-in-clothing/

http://www.biotecharticles.com/Toxicology-Article/Toxic-Fibers-and-Fabrics-699.html

http://bodyecology.com/articles/top_6_fabrics_you_should_avoid_wearing.php

https://www.choice.com.au/shopping/everyday-shopping/clothing/articles/chemicals-in-clothing

http://www.dailymail.co.uk/femail/article-2088623/Toxic-dyes-Lethal-logos-Cotton-drenched-formaldehyde--How-clothes-poison-you.html

http://www.drfranklipman.com/organic-fashion-should-we-worry-about-toxins-in-our-clothes/

http://easyhealthoptions.com/the-toxins-in-your-clothing/

http://fashionbi.com/newspaper/the-health-risks-of-toxic-fibers-and-fabrics

http://www.globalhealingcenter.com/natural-health/the-hidden-toxins-in-your-clothing/

http://www.greenpeace.org/international/en/publications/Campaign-reports/Toxics-reports/Big-Fashion-Stitch-Up/

http://www.mygutsy.com/are-your-childs-clothes-toxic/

http://www.naturalnews.com/037038_new_clothes_toxic_chemicals_washing.html

http://www.naturalnews.com/033436_toxic_chemicals_clothing.html

http://naturalsociety.com/chemical-clothing-toxic-chemicals-clothes-sick/

http://www.news18.com/news/india/cancer-causing-dyes-in-chinese-clothes-report-345310.html

http://theorganicsinstitute.com/organic/organic-clothing/

http://www.sixwise.com/newsletters/05/12/21/the-6-synthetic-fabrics-you-most-want-to-avoid-and-why.htm

http://www.viber.org.cn/en/html/news/2009/1241590561.html

Chapter Six:
http://www.badplastics.com/

http://www.breastcancerfund.org/clear-science/environmental-breast-cancer-links/plastics/

http://content.time.com/time/specials/packages/article/0,28804,1976909_1976908_1976938-4,00.html

http://www.dailymail.co.uk/health/article-2157423/Poisoned-plastic-Chemicals-water-bottles-food-packaging-linked-infertility-birth-defects-Scaremongering-truth.html

http://essentialstuff.org/index.php/2011/03/04/Cat/toxic-plastics-not-just-bpa/

http://healthwyze.org/reports/49-identifying-poisonous-plastics

http://www.healthychild.org/easy-steps/reduce-your-use-of-pvc-in-plastics-and-other-household-products/

http://io9.gizmodo.com/how-to-recognize-the-plastics-that-are-hazardous-to-you-461587850

http://articles.mercola.com/sites/articles/archive/2013/04/11/plastic-use.aspx

http://www.npr.org/2011/04/19/135245835/our-toxic-love-hate-relationship-with-plastics

http://www.oprah.com/health/The-Toxic-Chemicals-in-Plastic

http://www.realnatural.org/is-smelly-china-plastic-toxic/

http://www.smallfootprintfamily.com/avoiding-toxins-in-plastic

http://thesoftlanding.com/how-to-avoid-toxic-chemicals-in-food-containers-and-kitchen-appliances/

http://worldcentric.org/about-compostables/traditional-plastic/pollution

Chapter Seven:
http://www.cancer.gov/about-cancer/causes-prevention/risk/radiation/electromagnetic-fields-fact-sheet

http://www.cleanairyardcare.ca/sustainability/environmental-facts/

http://davidsuzuki.org/what-you-can-do/reduce-your-carbon-footprint/

https://www.edf.org/climate/cleanenergy

http://emwatch.com/emf-health-effects/

http://energy.gov/public-services/homes/heating-cooling

https://www3.epa.gov/climatechange/basics/

https://www3.epa.gov/carbon-footprint-calculator/

https://www.fix.com/blog/lawn-mowers-and-greener-lawn-care/

http://www.forbes.com/sites/houzz/2014/05/17/everything-you-need-to-know-about-adding-solar-panels-at-home/#313ec35b1862

http://www.theguardian.com/environment/2015/jan/07/much-worlds-fossil-fuel-reserve-must-stay-buried-prevent-climate-change-study-says

http://list25.com/25-ways-to-reduce-your-carbon-footprint/5/

http://mashable.com/2013/10/22/reduce-carbon-footprint/

http://www.motherearthnews.com/organic-gardening/gardening-techniques/sustainable-gardening-zm0z11zsto.aspx

http://www.ncbi.nlm.nih.gov/books/NBK11769/

http://www.niehs.nih.gov/health/topics/agents/air-pollution/

http://onescytherevolution.com/a-tale-of-two-scythes.html

https://www.osha.gov/SLTC/radiation/index.html

http://www.peoplepoweredmachines.com/faq-environment.htm

http://www.permaculture.co.uk/articles/owning-and-using-austrian-scythe

http://www.planetnatural.com/sustainable-gardening/

http://www.renewableenergyworld.com/index/tech.html

http://science.howstuffworks.com/environmental/green-tech/sustainable/5-solar-home.htm

http://science.howstuffworks.com/environmental/energy/geothermal-energy.htm

http://solarenergy.net/

http://www.sustainable-gardening.com/how-to/sustainable/practices

http://www.ucsusa.org/clean_energy/our-energy-choices/coal-and-other-fossil-fuels/the-hidden-cost-of-fossil.html

http://www.ucsusa.org/our-work/energy/our-energy-choices/our-energy-choices-renewable-energy

http://www.ucsusa.org/clean_energy/our-energy-choices/renewable-energy/how-geothermal-energy-works.html

http://www.wisegeek.org/what-is-clean-energy.htm

http://www.yourhome.gov.au/energy/heating-and-cooling

Chapter Eight:
http://bonfirehealth.com/adverse-effects-drugs-side-effects-toxic/

http://www.cancer.org/treatment/treatmentsandsideeffects/index

http://www.cdc.gov/vaccines/vac-gen/side-effects.htm

http://www.dailyrxnews.com/leukemia-risk-related-cancer-treatments

https://www.drugwatch.com/side-effects/

http://www.fda.gov/BiologicsBloodVaccines/Vaccines/def
ault.htm

http://healthcareforamericanow.org/2013/04/08/pharma-
711-billion-profits-price-gouging-seniors/

http://www.huffingtonpost.com/ethan-
rome/prescription-drug-companies-
pricing_b_2927900.html

http://www.kevinmd.com/blog/2012/01/physicians-
receive-adequate-training-nutrition.html

Lazarou J, Pomeranz BH, Corey PN. Incidence of adverse
drug reactions in hospitalized patients: A meta-analysis of
prospective studies. JAMA 1998;279:1200-1205. PubMed
Abstract Full Text

http://www.medicalnewstoday.com/info/cancer-oncology

http://www.medscape.com/viewarticle/830697#vp_2

http://articles.mercola.com/sites/articles/archive/2016/01
/26/whooping-cough-vaccine-ineffective.aspx

http://articles.mercola.com/sites/articles/archive/2015/11
/10/vaccine-injury-compensation.aspx

http://www.naturalnews.com/051608_price_gouging_fre
e_market_integrative_medicine.html

http://www.ncbi.nlm.nih.gov/pmc/articles/PMC1496869/

http://www.ninds.nih.gov/disorders/brain_basics/underst
anding_sleep.htm

http://www.pbs.org/newshour/rundown/need-15-
minutes-doctors-time/

http://www.philly.com/philly/blogs/healthcare/Drugs-
most-frequently-reported-for-adverse-reactions.html

http://blog.rphonthego.com/pharmacy-news/price-
gouging-pharmaceuticals/

http://www.vaccines.net/newpage114.htm

https://www.vaccines.gov/basics/safety/vaccine_ingredie
nts/index.html

http://vaxtruth.org/2011/08/vaccine-ingredients/

https://www.verywell.com/do-vaccines-cause-autism-
260121

http://www.webmd.com/sleep-disorders/features/sleep-hygiene

http://www.who.int/mediacentre/multimedia/podcasts/2009/lifestyle-interventions-20090109/en/

Willett, Walter C.; Koplan, Jeffrey P.; Nugent, Rachel; Dusenbury, Courtenay; Puska, Pekka; & Gaziano, Thomass. (2006). *Prevention of Chronic Disease by Means of Diet and Lifestyle Changes.* In T., Jamison Dean, G., Breman Joel, R., Measham Anthony, Alleyne, George, Claeson, Mariam, Evans, David B., Jha, Prabhat, Mills, Anne & Musgrove, Philip (Eds.), *Disease Control Priorities in Developing Countries* (pp. 833-850). Washington, D.C.: World Bank.

http://www.worstpills.org/public/page.cfm?op_id=4

Videos:

Food Inc.

Genetic Roulette

The Quest of the Cures...Continues, The Truth about Cancer